100 Questions & Answers About Osteoporosis and Osteopenia
Second Edition

Ivy M. Alexander, PhD, APRN,
ANP-BC, FAAN
Yale University School of Nursing

and

Karla A. Knight, RN, MSN
Health Care Writer

JONES AND BARTLETT PUBLISHERS
Sudbury, Massachusetts
BOSTON   TORONTO   LONDON   SINGAPORE

World Headquarters

Jones and Bartlett Publishers
40 Tall Pine Drive
Sudbury, MA 01776
978-443-5000
info@jbpub.com
www.jbpub.com

Jones and Bartlett Publishers
Canada
6339 Ormindale Way
Mississauga, Ontario L5V 1J2
Canada

Jones and Bartlett Publishers
International
Barb House, Barb Mews
London W6 7PA
United Kingdom

Jones and Bartlett's books and products are available through most bookstores and online booksellers. To contact Jones and Bartlett Publishers directly, call 800-832-0034, fax 978-443-8000, or visit our website, www.jbpub.com.

Substantial discounts on bulk quantities of Jones and Bartlett's publications are available to corporations, professional associations, and other qualified organizations. For details and specific discount information, contact the special sales department at Jones and Bartlett via the above contact information or send an email to specialsales@jbpub.com.

The authors, editor, and publisher have made every effort to provide accurate information. However, they are not responsible for errors, omissions, or for any outcomes related to the use of the contents of this book and take no responsibility for the use of the products and procedures described. Treatments and side effects described in this book may not be applicable to all people; likewise, some people may require a dose or experience a side effect that is not described herein. Drugs and medical devices are discussed that may have limited availability controlled by the Food and Drug Administration (FDA) for use only in a research study or clinical trial. Research, clinical practice, and government regulations often change the accepted standard in this field. When consideration is being given to use of any drug in the clinical setting, the health care provider or reader is responsible for determining FDA status of the drug, reading the package insert, and reviewing prescribing information for the most up-to-date recommendations on dose, precautions, and contraindications, and determining the appropriate usage for the product. This is especially important in the case of drugs that are new or seldom used.

Production Credits

Executive Publisher: Christopher Davis
Editorial Assistant: Sara Cameron
Associate Production Editor: Leah Corrigan
Senior Marketing Manager: Barb Bartoszek
Manufacturing and Inventory Supervisor:
  Amy Bacus

Composition: Glyph International
Cover Design: Carolyn Downer
Cover Images: © Thinkstock, © LiquidLibrary,
  © Photodisc, © Photos.com
Printing and Binding: Malloy, Inc.
Cover Printing: Malloy, Inc.

Library of Congress Cataloging-in-Publication Data
Alexander, Ivy M.
    100 questions & answers about osteoporosis and osteopenia/Ivy M. Alexander and Karla A. Knight.
      p. cm.
    Includes bibliographical references and index.
    ISBN 978-0-7637-7780-7 (alk. paper)
    1. Osteoporosis—Prevention—Popular works. 2. Osteopenia—Popular works. 3. Bones—Metabolism—Disorders—Popular works. 4. Osteoporosis—Miscellanea. I. Knight, Karla A. II. Title. III. Title: 100 questions and answers about osteoporosis and osteopenia. IV. Title: One hundred questions and answers about osteoporosis and osteopenia.
    RC931.O73A42 2010
    616.7'16—dc22   2009041695

6048
Printed in the United States of America
13 12 11 10 09   10 9 8 7 6 5 4 3 2 1

To our children:
Lauren, Gillian, Erin, Kyle, and Kelsey.
May you grow up and grow old with healthy bones.

Contents

Part 1: An Overview of Osteoporosis and Bone Development   1

Questions 1-10 describe the physiology of bone development and how osteoporosis and osteopenia occur, including:
- What is osteoporosis and what does it look like? How does osteopenia differ from osteoporosis?
- How does osteoporosis occur?
- Are there other vitamins and minerals that contribute to bone development?
- Which bones are affected by osteoporosis?

Part 2: Risk Factors and Testing   17

Questions 11-39 address the risk factors associated with osteoporosis, who should be tested, and how osteoporosis is diagnosed, including:
- Who gets osteoporosis?
- What are the risk factors for osteoporosis?
- How will I know if I have osteoporosis? Are there any signs or symptoms?
- How will my clinician use my test results to determine whether I have osteoporosis?

Part 3: Lifestyle Changes and Treatments   75

Questions 40-71 address lifestyle changes, exercise, calcium requirements and supplements, prescription medications, and other management strategies for osteoporosis and osteopenia, such as:
- I understand that exercise is important for the treatment of osteoporosis. Why?
- When should I take calcium supplements? Is there any particular time of day that makes calcium more effective? Should I take it before meals, with meals, or between meals?
- I know there are other vitamins and minerals that are important to bone development. Will I get enough of everything I need if I take a daily vitamin?
- Can I take prescription osteoporosis medications in combination with each other? Which medications could I use together to get more improvement in my bones?

What is osteoporosis? The simple answer is that it is the most prevalent bone disease in America and affects over 44 million people. Ten million Americans have osteoporosis; 34 million have low bone mass, which puts them at serious risk of osteoporosis. However, answers from many sources seem to perpetuate a series of myths about this disease. These myths include the following: osteoporosis is a normal consequence of aging; ONLY older white women develop osteoporosis; osteoporosis medication causes upset stomachs or that it always causes problems with the jaw (ONJ, or osteonecrosis of the jaw); taking calcium and vitamin D is enough to prevent osteoporosis; and exercise causes fractures in people with osteoporosis. Because these myths are so widely believed, people miss opportunities to prevent or treat bone loss.

How can we combat these damaging myths? First, research can show us what is true about osteoporosis. We now know that osteoporosis is—without a doubt—a disease, and not a part of normal aging. We also know that while many people who have osteoporosis are White, postmenopausal women, people of all races, both genders, and all adult ages can and do develop fragile bones. Recently published research also shows that the right kind of exercise builds bone, strengthens muscles, and prevents falls.

Second, we need to teach people the truth about bone loss. Despite the mention of osteoporosis in television shows and commercials, magazines, and newspapers, the American public remains woefully ignorant about it. Osteoporosis is a disease that starts in childhood and has consequences in later life. Kids today don't get enough calcium *or* exercise and are not achieving peak bone mass. Adolescent women who avoid calories and over-exercise for weight control stop their menses—again, a strong risk factor for inadequate bone development. Premenopausal women say, "I don't need to worry about that until menopause." Postmenopausal women say, "I can worry about that when I'm older." And older women and men who have low bone density, multiple fractures, and chronic pain say, "Why didn't someone tell me about this when it would have made a difference?"

The mission for many of us is to educate both the people who suffer from the debilitating consequences and those who are at risk of this disease. How can we teach them? We read, then listen, then read some more. This book, *100 Questions & Answers About Osteoporosis and Osteopenia, Second Edition*, is an excellent first step toward learning about osteoporosis. Read it cover to cover or look up the particular questions that interest you. Either way, this is a wonderful resource for all families.

Ivy Alexander and Karla Knight have written a treasure: a book that answers questions clearly, concisely, and accurately. They provide medication information, lists of risk factors, lifestyle issues that influence bone health as well as suggestions on how best to live with osteoporosis. They rely on the recent *Surgeon General's Report on Bone Health and Osteoporosis* (2004), recent research, and national organizations as sources for the most timely information on prevention and treatment of this bone disease. The message is clear: It is never too early or too late to prevent or treat osteoporosis. Anyone who reads *100 Questions & Answers About Osteoporosis and Osteopenia, Second Edition*, will know better than to believe the myths and old wives' tales that surround osteoporosis!

Deborah T. Gold, PhD
Associate Professor of Medical Sociology,
Departments of Psychiatry & Behavioral Sciences,
Sociology, and Psychology: Social & Health Sciences
Duke University Medical Center

Osteoporosis is the most common bone disease. When I was asked to co-author a second Jones and Bartlett book with Karla Knight, the first edition of this book focusing on osteoporosis, I was delighted to have the opportunity. I am again delighted to have the opportunity to work with Karla and update the information in this second edition. Many men and women still do not know about osteoporosis, the potentially devastating effects following osteoporosis-related fractures, and the many effective prevention and treatment options.

Osteoporosis is often considered a woman's disease, because of the dramatic increase in bone loss following menopause. But osteoporosis and osteopenia also affect men, young adults, and individuals with certain chronic illnesses or who take certain medications. The Surgeon General published a report on osteoporosis and osteopenia in 2004, highlighting the numbers of people affected by bone loss, the risks for bone loss, and the many options for preventing and treating bone loss. Yet so many remain unaware of these important facts.

My interest in osteopenia and osteoporosis stems from my clinical work, my research, and my own family history. I practice in internal medicine with a specialty in midlife women's health and have seen patients struggle with the after-effects of osteoporosis-related fractures. Through my research I have learned that many men and women are unaware of the risks of bone loss and the prevention strategies that can minimize bone loss. On a more personal level, my grandmother suffered with osteoporosis and experienced several broken bones during her older years, causing her significant pain and suffering. These facts continue to feed my interest in identifying and educating others about methods to prevent and manage osteoporosis. It is disturbing that so many of us are unaware of the needed vitamins and minerals to promote bone strength, and the exercises that can further assist in keeping healthy bones strong.

In this book, we describe the normal processes of bone turnover, the needed elements for healthy bone development, how to maintain healthy bones, and options for preventing and treating bone loss. All treatment options have some risks; it is our goal to provide you with understandable and accurate information, to provide a realistic picture that fairly portrays both the benefits and risks of various options, and to share information that you can use to make informed decisions about your own health. In addition to prescription medication options, we focus on the many lifestyle changes that you can adopt to help maintain your bone health and provide suggestions for supplements of essential minerals and vitamins as well. We have also included information regarding complementary and alternative options. Because we want to provide you with balanced and fair information about possible prevention and treatment options, we have included a section listing many of the references and resources that we used to write this book. Research information about specific strategies is an important part of understanding how well a specific strategy might work. We include this so that you can make informed decisions about prevention and treatment choices, and hope that you will read about future research as more information becomes available. We recognize that this book is one of many sources of information about osteoporosis. We encourage you to use it in addition to these other sources, talk with friends and family members, and consider carefully the many options that are available to you. And we hope you will use the information presented here in discussions with your clinicians.

The process of writing this book was really enjoyable. I am truly grateful to my co-author, Karla Knight. I appreciated our frequent conference calls and e-mail messages—the process has been exhilarating and exhausting at the same time!

Many people assisted us in making this book a reality. I owe special appreciation to the men and women who have shared their stories with me. Some of their stories are included in this book, using pseudonyms to protect their confidentiality. I am grateful to

Linda Bell, registered dietician; Dave Brzozowski and Mark Theriault, clinical pharmacists; and several other colleagues and friends who shared their expertise. I so appreciate the publishers at Jones and Bartlett—Chris Davis, Kathy Richardson, and Elizabeth Platt—who provided guidance and sage advice for the first edition and—Sara Cameron and Leah Corrigan—who have been instrumental in the writing of this second edition. I would never have completed this book without the encouragement of my many colleagues and friends. Most importantly I want to thank my family for their encouragement, support, and, most of all, understanding throughout this process.

—Ivy M. Alexander

Ivy Alexander and I had just finished writing *100 Questions & Answers About Menopause* when I was told I had bone loss. When my doctor told me that my T-score was in the osteopenia range, I was puzzled and upset. I felt like I had failed a test that I thought I was supposed to pass with flying colors. He immediately suggested a prescription medication. I countered with other options, but he said his experience was that if he did not treat patients with medication, they invariably came back with more bone loss the following year. Although I agreed to his plan, I wasn't entirely happy about it.

He also told me that if I didn't already ski or skate, I shouldn't put on skis or skates. I told him I worked out regularly and lifted weights two to three times a week. I had a good diet with plenty of calcium and Vitamin D. I wasn't small and thin. I was not a smoker, and I wasn't a heavy drinker. I don't take medications or have illnesses that are known to be tough on bones. I was still getting menstrual periods but they were very irregular, so I was still producing at least *some* estrogen. What was I doing wrong? I really, really, didn't want a bad grade on my test! Family and friends who know me well wouldn't be surprised that I considered my T-score tantamount to failing a homework assignment. My doctor said simply, "But you have a family history of osteoporosis. And that's a risk factor you can't change."

Since writing this book, I have tried to change my attitude toward my T-score. Without trying to sound like Pollyanna, I'm trying to see it as an opportunity to make some changes. Maybe I really wasn't taking enough calcium. And I certainly wasn't thinking very hard about Vitamin D. Maybe I wasn't really getting out there and exercising as much as I thought I was. In fact, our whole family has been using the local gym much more now, probably fearing some kind of lecture from me on the need for exercise!

I have also discovered that many friends and colleagues either have osteoporosis or are touched by it in some way. They may have family members who have it, or they know of someone with fractures at a younger age than expected.

My daughter Kelsey was very attentive to my comments and calculations about calcium. She even took calcium chewing gum to school to share with her high school friends and, of course, gave them my lecture about getting enough calcium every single day.

My son Kyle handed me the research that said that a beer a day helps build stronger bones. Now that's the kind of research I expect from a young adult just out of college! He did assure me that he was drinking milk and not beer every day.

My daughter Erin was a constant cheerleader for this book. She volunteered to get her bones checked at a bone screening in a local mall, even though in her mid-20s. She was probably the youngest person to sign up!

Tom, ever the supportive husband, how could I write at home without you? You're great about sharing our one computer so that I can write. And I count my blessings every day that you always find the time to do the laundry and the dishes, with never a resentful glance in my direction.

My mom's experience with osteoporosis continued to inspire me while writing this book. I hope I'll be able to stay active and keep my sense of humor the way she has. My dad went to the post office at least once a week for the past 6 months to send me osteoporosis information from my mom. Thanks, Mom and Dad!

I could never have written the first edition of this book without the support of my neighbor and friend, Kathy Richardson.

Her experience as an Associate Editor, and that of Executive Publisher Chris Davis, and Special Projects Editor Elizabeth Platt, helped me immeasurably. For this second edition, I thank Editorial Assistant Sara Cameron and Associate Production Editor Leah Corrigan for their organization skills and helpful e-mails!

Special thanks to Bertha Earp; Joan C. Borgatti, RN, MEd; Gilbert Carley, DMD; Mona Vogel, RPh; Jeff Robichaud, BA, DC; Barry Bailey, MS, CLMT; Karen McCarte, CPNP; and the late Dorothy Sexton, EdD, RN, for their advice and input for this book.

Ivy, thank you for being such a great co-author, especially when you had so many other professional responsibilities as a researcher, practitioner, and educator. I will miss our weekly conversations about our books and all the other things we managed to talk about!

And to other friends and colleagues, thanks for listening to me through the writing of yet another book. Your support and friendship mean everything to me.

—Karla A. Knight

Introduction

PART ONE

An Overview of Osteoporosis and Bone Development

What is osteoporosis and what does it look like?

How does osteopenia differ from osteoporosis?

If we "lose bone," where does it go? Can it be replaced once it's lost?

More...

1. What is osteoporosis and what does it look like? How does osteopenia differ from osteoporosis?

Osteoporosis is a disease in which bones become less dense, lose strength, and are more likely to break (**fracture**). Some people describe bones with osteoporosis as "Swiss cheese." The word osteoporosis is derived from the Greek *osteo*, meaning bones, and *porosis*, meaning with holes. Osteoporosis happens mainly to women at midlife and later, but also can happen to men and children. In children, new bone forms more quickly than it breaks down so that bone is actually growing all the time. In adults, bone goes through a constant and normal process where new bone is formed and old bone is broken down simultaneously and at relatively even rates. When more bone is lost than is being formed, osteopenia and osteoporosis develop. **Figure 1** compares normal bone with osteoporotic bone.

Although the words sound somewhat alike, osteoporosis and osteopenia are a little different from one another.

Osteoporosis

In Greek, literally meaning bones (osteo) with holes (porosis); a disease in which bones become less dense, lose strength, and are more likely to break (fracture).

Fracture

To break, splinter, or crack a bone.

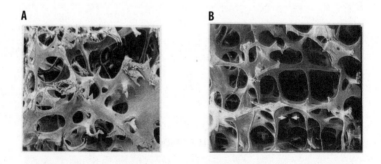

A   **B**

Figure 1   Comparison of normal bone with osteoporosis. A. Normal bone. B. Osteoporotic bone. Courtesy of the National Association of Nurse Practitioners in Women's Health (NPWH). From Dempster DW et al. *J Bone Miner Res* 1986;1:15–21.

Both relate to bone loss, but the difference is in how much bone is lost. **Osteopenia**, like osteoporosis, means that the process of bone development has become unbalanced and the rate of bone loss exceeds the rate of new bone growth. With osteopenia, some bone has been lost but not as much as with osteoporosis. Although osteopenia increases your risk of breaking a bone, the risk is not as high as it is with osteoporosis. The word osteopenia comes from two Greek words: *osteo*, which literally means "bone," and *penia*, which means "lacking." So osteopenia is a milder version of osteoporosis but is still very important to your understanding of bone health. Many people with osteopenia will go on to develop osteoporosis. Some clinicians prefer to use the term "low bone mass" instead of osteopenia.

2. Why is it important to know about osteoporosis and osteopenia?

Osteoporosis is the most common bone disease. While osteoporosis and osteopenia are painless, it is still important for you to understand how they affect your personal health, family, finances, and lifestyle. A recent report from the U.S. Surgeon General says that by 2020, half of all Americans over the age of 50 will be at risk for fractures as a result of osteoporosis. Current estimates indicate that osteoporosis is an expensive healthcare problem, costing Americans $18 billion per year.

Osteoporosis is costly not only in dollars and cents, but also in terms of poor health, **disability**, and social isolation. Fractures that result from osteoporosis can be devastating. Up to 20% of those who fracture a hip will die within 1 year of the fracture.

Osteopenia

In Greek, literally meaning bone (osteo) that is lacking (penia); the process of bone development has become unbalanced and the rate of bone loss exceeds the rate of new bone growth. With osteopenia, some bone has been lost but not as much as with osteoporosis.

Disability

A physical or mental impairment that causes inability to perform normal or routine activities.

Overview and Bone Development

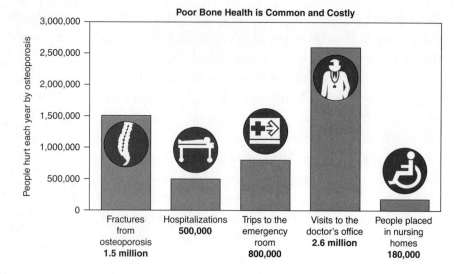

Figure 2   Impact of osteoporosis. Courtesy of the U.S. Department of Health and Human Services, *The 2004 Surgeon General's Report on Bone Health and Osteoporosis. What it means to you.* Washington, DC: Office of the Surgeon General; 2004.

Of those who survive, 50% will not be able to return to independent living. Those who suffer fractures as a result of osteoporosis may not be able to dress themselves or carry on other activities of daily living, frequently causing depression and isolation from others. About 20% will need nursing home or assisted living care after a hip fracture because they are not able to live independently. **Figure 2** shows the impact of poor bone health and why it's important for you to be aware of osteoporosis.

3. How does osteoporosis occur?

Osteoporosis, or bone loss, occurs when the process of bone breakdown and bone formation gets out of balance. The cells that cause bone breakdown (**osteoclasts**) start to make canals and holes in the

Osteoclast

Type of cell that causes bone breakdown.

4

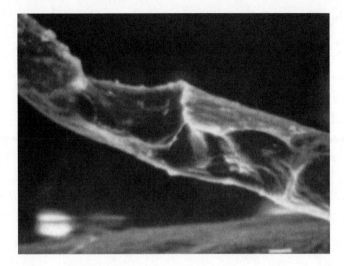

Figure 3   Microscopic view of osteoporotic bone. Courtesy of the National Association of Nurse Practitioners in Women's Health (NPWH).

bone faster than the cells that cause bone formation (**osteoblasts**) can make new bone to fill in the holes. The bone becomes fragile and more likely to break. **Figure 3** shows a microscopic view of weak bone and surrounding holes.

Osteoblast

Type of cell that causes bone formation.

When bone has to give up some of its calcium to ensure that blood levels of calcium stay normal, bone is weakened by the loss of calcium. The weakening of bone by its loss of calcium also leads to osteopenia and osteoporosis.

Taking in extra calcium and vitamin D alone will not prevent osteoporosis. Because of the way bone develops, the mechanical stress on bone caused by exercise is also important for preventing osteoporosis. The less you exercise, the less the osteoblasts work to make new bone. You need both weight-bearing and **resistive exercise** to promote strong bones (see Questions 42 and 43).

Resistive exercise

Type of activity that pushes and pulls muscles to strengthen them; examples are swimming, biking, and weight-lifting.

5

When the body has not formed adequate bone during childhood and young adulthood, the lack of **bone mass** is also termed osteoporosis or osteopenia, depending on how frail the bones are. Even if your bones are not so frail that you have osteopenia or osteoporosis, not reaching peak bone mass in your youth makes osteoporosis more likely to occur. The reason that building strong bones in childhood is so important is that if a young adult does not have peak bone mass, osteoporosis is more likely to develop despite preventive measures taken later in life.

4. How is bone made? Do we stop making bone when we become adults?

The 206 bones of the human body are important for their ability to support surrounding tissue and muscles, protect the body's organs, allow movement, manufacture blood cells, and provide storage for calcium and phosphorus, minerals that are released from the bone when needed. Given bone's many functions, it's not surprising that bone development is a complicated process.

Each bone is made up of **collagen**, which is a protein substance, and minerals such as calcium and phosphorus. This matrix of soft and hard elements gives bone its versatility in being able to support the weight and movement of the body, while also storing vital calcium for the normal functioning of muscles and nerves.

In infancy, the process of hardening the **cartilage** that we're born with begins. **Bone modeling** is a process that takes place in childhood and adolescence. It is the development of new bone at one site and the destruction of old bone at another site within the same bone at the

Bone mass

The volume, density, or quantity of bone.

Collagen

A protein substance used by osteoblasts to make new bone and keep teeth strong. Also found in connective tissue such as skin, tendons, and ligaments throughout the body.

Cartilage

Rubbery connective tissue that is found in joints and the outer ear.

Bone modeling

A process that takes place in childhood and adolescence where new bone is developed at one site and old bone is destroyed at another site within the same bone at the same time.

same time. The amount of new bone that is developed exceeds the amount of old bone that is broken down. This process is the way in which **peak bone mass** (the maximum amount of bone) is achieved, usually in our early 20s to 30s, and also allows the bones of childhood to develop at different rates and shift in space, until the adult skeleton is fully formed.

Yes, we continue to make bone as adults in a continuous process called **bone <u>re</u>modeling**. Bone-resorbing cells (osteoclasts) secrete enzymes, which digest bone and create holes. Bone-forming cells (osteoblasts) migrate to the bone surface and, by secreting a particular type of collagen, fill in the holes. Unlike the process in childhood, the osteoblasts do not function independently. Instead, they act in response to the activity of the osteoclasts and stresses on bone, such as exercise. **Figure 4** shows the process of remodeling. In response to the hole-making activity of the osteoclasts, the osteoblasts help to form new bone to fill in the holes.

Peak bone mass

The maximum amount of bone.

Bone remodeling

A process in adults where bone is constantly made. Bone resorbing cells (osteoclasts) secrete enzymes that digest bone and create holes. Bone forming cells (osteoblasts) migrate to the bone surface and, by secreting a particular type of collagen, fill in the holes.

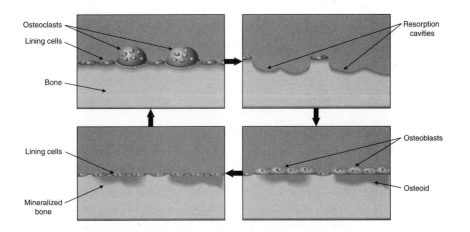

Osteoclasts
Lining cells
Bone
Resorption cavities
Lining cells
Mineralized bone
Osteoblasts
Osteoid

Figure 4 **The bone remodeling process. Courtesy of Eli Lilly and Company.**

Overview and Bone Development

Calcium, phosphate, and other substances mix with water, somewhat like cement, and harden the collagen, which has been laid down in a matrix-type pattern. As we age, the process of bone remodeling does not stop, but it does slow down. Our bones are very busy—we recycle our entire skeleton about every 10 years!

We recycle our entire skeleton about every 10 years!

Osteoclasts and osteoblasts are found in all bone, but are found in greater numbers in the hip, spine, and "long" bones of the thigh (femur), upper arms (humerus), lower legs (tibia and fibula), and lower arms (radius and ulna). This is why the most accurate measurements of bone density are taken from the hip and spine, rather than the smaller bones of the hands and feet.

5. If we "lose bone," where does it go? Can it be replaced once it's lost?

We usually don't begin to lose bone until we are in our mid-30s, which is after our peak bone mass has been reached. Around this age, the process of remodeling takes over and the balancing act of replacing lost bone with new bone begins.

If you do not continually take in enough of the nutrient building blocks for bones, such as protein, calcium, and vitamin D, and if you do not get appropriate exercise, the process of remodeling becomes unbalanced. If the osteoclasts outpace the osteoblasts during remodeling, holes will be made faster than they can be filled by the osteoblasts. The osteoclasts break down collagen, which is excreted in urine, and in this way bone is lost. When calcium and phosphorus are taken from the bones in your body to replace low levels of calcium and phosphorus in the blood, bone loss also occurs.

Once bone is lost, it can be replaced. However, increasing bone mass once it has been lost requires the right combination of exercise, intake of essential nutrients, and, often, **prescription medications** (see Part Three).

6. What roles do calcium and vitamin D play in developing bones?

Calcium and vitamin D play vital roles in bone development. Once the osteoblasts have secreted the collagen to fill in the holes made by the osteoclasts, the collagen is strengthened by **lysine** (an amino acid) and hardened with calcium, giving bone its hardness and strength. The strengthening of the new collagen takes place over a 1- to 2-week period.

Most **calcium** in the body is stored in bone. In fact, bone is 40% calcium. When blood levels of calcium dip below normal, calcium is taken from the bone to restore normal blood levels. The body loses calcium through urine, sweat, and stool, and because it is constantly excreted, you must always take in enough calcium to maintain normal blood levels. Keeping your blood calcium at normal levels prevents the bone from releasing its stores of calcium, thus protecting your bone strength.

Vitamin D is necessary for the absorption of calcium and phosphorus from the intestinal tract. If your body has inadequate vitamin D, calcium and phosphorus will not be absorbed from your intestines but instead will be taken from your bones, regardless of how much calcium you are taking in. Vitamin D is also important

Prescription medications

An instruction from a health care professional who is licensed to provide written authorization for medications or devices to be issued by a pharmacy.

Lysine

An amino acid that strengthens collagen in bone formation.

Calcium

A mineral necessary for the body to thrive; bone is made up of 40% calcium. When calcium in the blood is low, it is taken from bone. The body loses calcium through urine, sweat, and stool, and it must be replaced through intake of certain foods and exercise.

Vitamin D

A type of vitamin that is necessary for the absorption of calcium and phosphorus from the intestinal tract.

Calcitriol

A hormone resulting from the conversion of vitamin D by liver and kidney enzymes to aid in balancing the activity of the osteoclasts and osteoblasts.

Osteomalacia

A disease character-
ized by a gradual
softening and bend-
ing of the bones with
varying severity of
pain; often comes
from a vitamin D
deficiency; may also
be called "adult
rickets."

Vitamin A

Helps to regulate
osteoclast and
osteoblast activities in
bone modeling and
remodeling; too much
of it disrupts these
processes.

Vitamin B_6

Indirectly helps with
bone development by
lowering levels of
homocysteine, a body
substance associated
with fractures due to
osteoporosis; high
homocysteine levels
may increase the risk
of heart disease.

Homocysteine

A substance associ-
ated with fractures
due to osteoporosis
as well as heart dis-
ease; can be reduced
by eating a diet high
in folic acid (e.g.,
green leafy vegeta-
bles and fruits) or
by taking vitamins
B_6 and B_{12}.

for bone strength because it is transformed into a hormone called **calcitriol** by liver and kidney enzymes to
aid in balancing the activity of the bone-forming cells
(osteoblasts) and bone breakdown cells (osteoclasts). If
you are severely deficient in vitamin D, you may
develop **osteomalacia** ("softened" bones), which can
result in bone pain, leg deformities, and fractures. So
it is important to consistently get adequate vitamin D,
either from supplements or from foods.

7. Are there other vitamins and minerals that contribute to bone development?

In addition to vitamin D, the following vitamins play a
role in bone health:

- **Vitamin A** plays an essential role in developing
  healthy bones by helping to regulate osteoclast and
  osteoblast activities in bone modeling and remodeling, but too much of it can actually damage your
  bones by disrupting these processes.
- **Vitamin B_6** indirectly helps with bone development
  by lowering levels of **homocysteine,** a body substance
  associated with fractures due to osteoporosis. High
  homocysteine levels may also increase your risk of
  heart disease.
- **Vitamin C** is important for bone development because
  of its role in making collagen, which is one of the
  substances secreted by the osteoblasts to fill in the
  holes or cavities in bone.
- Although you might associate **vitamin K** with
  blood clotting, it also plays a role in bone growth
  because it aids in the production of **osteocalcin,**
  another protein that is part of the process of bone

remodeling. Vitamin K can also help prevent bone from being broken down and calcium from being excreted in urine. Research is currently under way studying the long-term effects of vitamin K on bones. Getting insufficient amounts of vitamin K may lead to an increase in the risk of hip fracture.

- **Folate**, or folic acid, is a vitamin known to prevent spinal defects in developing fetuses, and like vitamin B_6 is also important in reducing homocysteine levels; high homocysteine levels have been associated with an increase in osteoporosis-related fractures.

Calcium is probably the most well known mineral associated with bone health. However, magnesium and phosphorus play important roles as well. **Magnesium** and **phosphorus** contribute to the hardening of the bone in the process of remodeling. If your blood becomes too acidic, calcium can be taken from your bones. It is speculated that magnesium works with potassium to make blood less acidic and therefore less likely to take calcium from bones. Fluoride, boron, copper, manganese, and sodium are all minerals that contribute to forming healthy bones as well (see Question 53).

8. Are there other substances that affect bone development? What about hormones?

Bone development is a complicated process and requires many different substances and hormones, even a specific gene. Scientists have discovered that there is a gene that is required for the formation of the body's skeleton. If this gene is not present in the embryo stage of development, bones cannot form correctly.

Vitamin C

Important for bone development because of its role in making collagen, which is one of the substances secreted by the osteoblasts to fill in the holes or cavities in bone.

Vitamin K

Associated with blood clotting, it helps in the production of osteocalcin, another protein that is part of the process of bone remodeling; this vitamin also helps to prevent bone from being broken down and calcium from being excreted in urine.

Osteocalcin

A type of protein that is part of the bone remodeling process.

Folate

A vitamin known to prevent spinal defects in developing fetuses; also important in reducing homocysteine levels, which have been associated with an increase in osteoporosis-related fractures.

Magnesium

An alkaline earth element that contributes to the hardening of the bone in the process of remodeling.

Phosphorus

A salt or ester of phosphoric acid that contributes to the hardening of the bone in the process of remodeling.

Calcitonin

A hormone naturally secreted by the thyroid gland that binds with osteoclasts, making them less active and allowing the osteoblasts to form more bone.

Parathyroid hormone (PTH)

Secreted by the parathyroid glands (located by the thyroid gland), PTH assists in the regulation of calcium by promoting the absorption of calcium from the intestine and reducing loss of calcium from the urine by the kidney; excessive amounts can lead to bone loss.

Cortisol

Secreted by the adrenal glands (located by the kidneys); is needed in small amounts for bone growth. Large amounts of cortisol can interfere with bone growth. The synthetic form of cortisol, or steroids, used in the treatment of some diseases, can cause bone loss.

In addition to this gene, the following other substances and hormones are needed for normal bone formation:

- **Calcitonin**, a hormone naturally secreted by the thyroid gland (located in the neck), binds with the osteoclasts, making them less active, which allows the osteoblasts to form more bone.
- **Parathyroid hormone (PTH)**, secreted by the parathyroid glands (located by the thyroid gland), assists in the regulation of calcium by promoting the absorption of calcium from the intestine and reducing loss of calcium from the urine by the kidney. Interestingly, while PTH is necessary and important at normal levels, excessive amounts can lead to bone loss.
- **Cortisol**, secreted by the adrenal glands (located by the kidneys), is needed in small amounts for bone growth. Large amounts of cortisol can interfere with bone growth. The synthetic form of cortisol, or steroids, used in the treatment of some diseases (see Question 15), can cause bone loss.
- **Growth hormone**, secreted by the pituitary gland (located in the brain), is important to both bone formation and bone **resorption** (destruction of the bone) but is most important in its role of increasing the speed of bone formation during puberty.
- **Thyroid hormones**, secreted by the thyroid gland, regulate the body's metabolism and help to control the rate at which bone remodeling occurs. However, too much thyroid hormone (hyperthyroidism) can cause excessive bone destruction.
- **Insulin,** a hormone secreted by the pancreas to help the body use carbohydrates and sugar, and **leptin,** a newly identified hormone that is found in fat cells, both have effects on bone growth.
- **Sex hormones,** such as **estrogen** and **testosterone,** are important for bone growth and for maintaining

bone mass. The estrogen produced in adolescents at the end of puberty is important for closing the bone growth plates, which prevents further growth in height. Estrogen and testosterone, both produced in men and women, stimulate bone formation. Testosterone also aids in muscle growth, which increases the mechanical stress on bones, which in turn encourages more bone formation by the osteoblasts.

9. What does menopause have to do with osteoporosis? Are there different kinds of osteoporosis?

There are actually two types of osteoporosis: primary osteoporosis and secondary osteoporosis. Either type can affect men, women, and children. **Primary osteoporosis** is age-related and affects women more severely and earlier in life than men. **Secondary osteoporosis** is caused by other disease processes or medications used to treat various diseases or problems. Secondary osteoporosis is also more common in women because the illnesses that cause bone loss or the problems that require medications that affect bone remodeling more often affect women.

Primary osteoporosis, although occurring in both men and women, is age-related and tends to occur mostly in women and about 10 years earlier than in men. This is because the rate of bone loss is different in women than in men. Women rapidly lose bone in the 4 to 8 years after menopause, and then continue with a slower rate of bone loss like men, who also experience bone loss over many years. Bone loss from primary osteoporosis is most common in the hip, but can affect all bones in the body.

Growth hormone

Secreted by the pituitary gland (located in the brain); is important to both bone formation and bone resorption (destruction of the bone), but is most important in its role of increasing the speed of bone formation during puberty.

Resorption

Process by the osteoclasts of breaking down bone.

Thyroid hormones

Hormones secreted by the thyroid gland that regulate the body's metabolism and help to control the rate at which bone remodeling occurs.

Insulin

A hormone secreted by the pancreas to help the body use carbohydrates and sugar; has effects on bone growth.

Leptin

A hormone found in fat cells that has effects on bone growth.

Sex hormones

Hormones such as estrogen and testosterone that are important for bone growth and for maintaining bone mass.

Estrogen

A hormone secreted by the ovaries in women and in body tissues in both women and men.

Testosterone

A hormone formed by the testes in males and, to a far lesser degree, by the ovary and adrenal glands in women; important for normal sexual development and function in both men and women.

Primary osteoporosis

A bone disease that is age-related; affects women more severely and earlier in life than men.

Secondary osteoporosis

Caused by other disease processes or medications used to treat various diseases or problems.

Menopause

The specific point in time in women occurring after 12 consecutive months without a menstrual period that does not have another identifiable cause, such as illness or medication.

Primary osteoporosis affects the entire skeleton, particularly in women following menopause. Natural **menopause** is medically defined as the specific point in time occurring after 12 consecutive months without a menstrual period that does not have another identifiable cause, such as illness or medication. **Postmenopause**, the time following menopause, is when many women develop osteoporosis. The decrease in bone mass in postmenopausal women is a direct result of the loss of estrogen. Menopause for any reason (e.g., surgery, chemotherapy) can cause bone loss.

Postmenopausal women lose about 2% and sometimes even up to 5% of their bone mass per year for the first 4 to 8 years following menopause. Twenty percent of their total bone loss takes place in those first 4 to 8 years after menopause. The majority of White women can expect to have osteopenia or osteoporosis once they have been in postmenopause for 10 years.

Because primary osteoporosis is caused mostly by estrogen loss in women, one of the preventive treatments for primary osteoporosis in women is **estrogen therapy (ET)**. Estrogen (with or without progesterone) is usually prescribed to prevent osteoporosis only if the woman also has significant other symptoms of menopause such as **hot flashes** and **night sweats**. When estrogen therapy is used for the relief of menopause symptoms, it is called **menopause hormone therapy (MHT)**. If you have a uterus, progesterone must be added to the estrogen therapies (see Question 64). An estrogen patch is also available to prevent the bone loss associated with postmenopause. Recent studies indicate that this patch effectively reduces hot flashes as well (see Question 65).

10. Which bones are affected by osteoporosis?

Although the hipbones and the **vertebrae** (bones of the spine) provide the best measurements of bone loss, osteoporosis occurs in all bones. The osteoblasts and osteoclasts are most active in the bones of the body's central region—that is, bones of the hip and vertebrae—and the **long bones** of the arms and legs. The skull bone is very rarely affected by osteoporosis.

Fractures of the hip and vertebrae are also the most common fractures. Because all bones can be affected by osteoporosis, clinicians usually recommend that individuals with weakened bones, like those caused by osteoporosis and osteopenia, avoid playing certain sports or engaging in certain activities that will increase the likelihood of falls which, of course, increase the risk of fractures of any bones, but particularly the hip (see Question 44).

Every bone has a soft inner portion known as the bone marrow as well as an outer portion made up of **trabecular bone** (connective spongy bone tissue) and **cortical bone** (the hard outer shell). Trabecular bone makes up the softer inner shell of all bones and is present in higher amounts in the hip, vertebrae, wrists, and ends of the long bones. The **central** and long bones have more trabecular bone than the other smaller bones in the body. Trabecular bone, which comprises about 20% of the body's bone, provides strength and integrity, produces blood products, and provides the surface used for mineral exchange, such as phosphorus and calcium. Bone marrow is found in the spaces between trabecular bone. Cortical bone makes up the hard outer shell of bone and is critical for bone strength. **Figure 5** shows trabecular and cortical bone.

Postmenopause

The time following menopause, when women rapidly lose bone and may develop osteoporosis.

Estrogen therapy (ET)

Estrogen-containing products used in the treatment of peri-menopausal and menopausal symptoms. Estrogen taken for this purpose is called MHT (menopause hormone therapy).

Hot flashes

Sensations of heat, occurring during perimenopause and often well into post-menopause, that begin at the head and spread over the entire body.

Night sweats

Sweating that occurs at night resulting from hot flashes during perimenopause and postmenopause.

Menopause hormone therapy (MHT)

Type of treatment used for the relief of menopause symptoms; also helps to prevent bone loss.

Vertebrae

Individual bones of the spine. Fractures of these bones are the most common fractures in people with osteoporosis.

Long bones

The larger bones of the legs (femur, tibia, fibula) and arms (humerus, ulna, radius).

Trabecular bone

Connective spongy tissue of bone, particularly of the central and long bones. Provides strength and integrity, houses bone marrow, produces blood products, and provides the surface used for the exchange of calcium and phosphorus.

Cortical bone

The hard outer shell of bone; critical for bone strength.

Central bones

Bones that are found in the main or central areas of the body, such as the hips, vertebrae, and spine. These bones provide the best measures for determining bone mineral density.

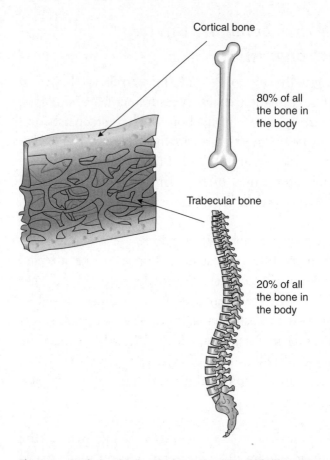

Cortical bone

80% of all the bone in the body

Trabecular bone

20% of all the bone in the body

Figure 5   Cortical and trabecular bone. Courtesy of Eli Lilly and Company, Einhorn TA, The Bone Organ System in: Osteoporosis. Eds. Marcus et al. Academic Press 1996.

In primary osteoporosis, women lose 5% to 10% of cortical bone and 20% to 30% of trabecular bone during the rapid bone loss occurring in the 4 to 8 years following menopause. In contrast, men and women (after the faster postmenopausal bone loss) experience a slower rate of bone loss as a result of aging. Occurring slowly over many years, this type of bone loss accounts for about a 20% to 25% loss of both cortical and trabecular bone. Thus, women are at risk for much greater bone loss than men.

PART TWO

Risk Factors and Testing

Who gets osteoporosis?

Could I be taking any medications that affect bone health?

Can my clinician tell if I have osteoporosis during my annual check-up?

More...

11. Who gets osteoporosis?

Both men and women can develop osteoporosis. Although more people with osteoporosis are women, particularly those who are postmenopausal, about 2 million men in the United States currently have osteoporosis, and one out of four will experience a fracture related to osteoporosis in his lifetime.

Primary osteoporosis, which occurs in both men and women, is a result of aging. It occurs most frequently in postmenopausal women due to the rapid loss in bone associated with the normal drop in estrogen around menopause. The average age of menopause in the United States is 51. The World Health Organization (WHO) reports that 35% of postmenopausal White women have osteoporosis. Primary osteoporosis or age-related osteoporosis tends to develop toward the end of life in men. The American Academy of Orthopedic Surgeons reports that almost 14% of men over the age of 85 have osteoporosis, while only 2% of men between the ages of 65 and 74 have osteoporosis.

Secondary osteoporosis, which occurs as a result of medications or diseases that cause bone loss, can also occur in both men and women, at any age. Since more women than men have the medical conditions treated with the class of drugs known as glucocorticoids and other medications that cause bone loss, this type of osteoporosis occurs more frequently in women.

White and Asian women develop osteoporosis more frequently than their Hispanic and Black counterparts. White men are also at higher risk for developing osteoporosis than Hispanic and Black men. There are few data available on Asian men and osteoporosis, but like Asian women, Asian men are likely at greater risk than Hispanic and Black men.

Postmenopausal women and men in later life are not the only ones who experience osteoporosis and osteopenia. Children, adolescents, and young adults can get osteoporosis too, particularly those with genetic or nutritional disorders and those with eating disorders such as **anorexia nervosa** and **bulimia,** because they do not make hormones or absorb calcium, vitamin D, and other nutrients and protein required for normal bone development. Those who are treated with medications that interfere with bone development may also get osteoporosis. People who are treated with long-term methotrexate (>1 month), usually for cancer or arthritis, are more at risk. Long-term use of the gonadotropin-releasing hormone analogs, such as Lupron® for the treatment of **endometriosis** in young women, can contribute to the development of osteoporosis as well. The most common class of medication to cause osteoporosis or osteopenia at any age is corticosteroids, used for such problems as lupus, arthritis, or asthma. Osteoporosis occurring after taking a glucocorticoid is so common that it has its own name: **glucocorticoid-induced osteoporosis (GIO).**

The more risk factors you have, the more likely it is that you will develop osteoporosis. Question 12 has a list of risk factors.

Maggie's comment:

When I went for my annual gynecology check-up at around the age of 52, my gynecologist asked me, as usual, if my family history of medical conditions had changed. His ears perked up when I told him that my mother had been diagnosed with spinal stenosis. When I looked back, I remembered

Anorexia nervosa

A disorder characterized by fear of becoming obese, thinking the body is larger than it really is, severe weight loss, and an aversion to food. Once thought to only affect teenage girls, it is now recognized in women of all ages and rarely in men.

Bulimia

An eating disorder that usually includes episodes of binge eating (eating very large amounts of food) and purging (inducing vomiting or diarrhea to get food out of the system).

Endometriosis

A painful condition characterized by the abnormal presence of endometrial (uterine lining) tissue outside the uterus, such as on the ovary, colon, or bladder.

Glucocorticoid-induced osteoporosis (GIO)

A type of osteoporosis that develops in people of all ages who are on glucocorticoid drug therapy.

that my dad had an unusual fracture of his collarbone when he was about 72, and for the last 10 years of his life he had a very stooped appearance.

My doctor said that I should have a bone density test to determine if I had osteoporosis in my hip or spine. My test did show some bone loss in my hip. I was angry because I had no symptoms whatsoever and believed that I was taking good care of my health.

When I was first diagnosed with bone loss, I told my two younger brothers about it. My brothers were tested for osteoporosis but did not have it. Their doctors, however, were careful to note that they have a family history of bone loss.

12. What are the risk factors for osteoporosis?

Unless you break a bone, osteoporosis is painless.

Unless you break a bone, osteoporosis is painless. It's therefore important to know if you are at risk for developing it. While men and women have many of the same risk factors for osteoporosis and osteopenia, a few are gender-specific. The following factors put you at risk for osteopenia and osteoporosis:

- *Age.* Bone mass decreases as you age. So as you get older, you are more likely to develop osteoporosis. While osteoporosis can affect women and men at any age, it most commonly affects postmenopausal women and older men. The National Osteoporosis Foundation reports that 75% of all cases of osteoporosis are diagnosed in White women over the age of 50. As men age, they too can develop osteoporosis, and it's much more likely to occur in men who are well into late life.

- *Gender.* Eighty percent of those with osteoporosis are women. Although men account for approximately 20% of cases, they develop osteoporosis much later if they get primary osteoporosis. Men can develop secondary osteoporosis much earlier in life as a result of medications or illness, however. Women are at greater risk because they start with less bone mass and lose it over time at a faster rate than men.

- *Race.* If you are White, particularly of Northern European descent, or Asian, you are at higher risk for osteoporosis than if you are Hispanic or Black. In fact, 65% of Black women have low bone mineral density. But if you are Black, you are still at significant risk—10% of Black women have osteoporosis. Over 300,000 Black women have osteoporosis, and approximately 90% of the fractures sustained by older Black women are due to osteoporosis. As Black women age, their risk for fracture doubles every 7 years, and the mortality rates following hip fractures are greater among Black than White women. Similarly, older White males are also more likely to get osteoporosis than their Black or Hispanic counterparts.

- *Fracture history.* If you have broken a bone in adulthood (about 50 years of age or older), you are more likely to have reduced bone mass and therefore osteoporosis. This is particularly important if the fracture occurred with a low amount of trauma or force.

- *Family history.* If you have a first-degree relative (mother, father, brother, sister, son, daughter) with osteoporosis or osteopenia, you are more at risk for bone loss.

- *Poor health.* Frailty and **dementia** are both associated with lower bone mass.

Women are at greater risk because they start with less bone mass and lose it over time at a faster rate than men.

Dementia

Condition marked by memory loss, lack of ability to attend to personal care, personality changes, impaired reasoning, and bouts of disorientation.

- *Cigarette smoking.* Nicotine in cigarettes causes problems with bone formation by interfering with the important role of estrogen and testosterone in bone development.
- *Excessive alcohol intake.* Heavy drinking interferes with calcium absorption as well as the osteoblast activity in bone formation. Ironically, two beers per day for men and two glasses of wine per day for women have been associated with increased bone mineral density. However, more alcohol than this increases your risk of osteoporosis instead of your bone mineral density.
- *Excessive caffeine intake.* It's not entirely clear exactly how caffeine affects your risk for osteoporosis. One study found that the risk of hip fracture was increased if more than two cups of coffee or four cups of tea were consumed per day. In other studies, coffee and tea consumption was not associated with lower bone density or fracture. In fact, one of these studies found that tea consumption was associated with higher bone density. Conflicting study results aside, moderate caffeine intake (1–2 servings of caffeinated beverages per day) is not likely to affect your bones if you get adequate calcium and vitamin D. The following substances contain the most caffeine:

  - Coffee (8 ounces, brewed): about 135 mg (depends on strength and process of brewing)
  - Caffeinated tea (8 ounces): about 50 to 70 mg (depends on how long it is steeped)
  - Coca-Cola (12 ounces): about 34.5 mg
  - Diet Coke (12 ounces): 46.5 mg

  You should also be aware that if you are drinking lots of coffee, tea, and soda, you are likely drinking fewer of the calcium-rich beverages such as milk and orange juice.

- *Excessive soda intake.* While phosphorus is needed for normal bone development, too much of it can cause bone loss. More than 3000 to 4000 milligrams (mg) of phosphorus per day puts you at increased risk. It was once thought that soda (pop, tonic, carbonated beverages other than water) contained excessive amounts of phosphoric acid; however, a caffeinated cola drink contains only about 50 mg of phosphorus. The more important issue is that you may be drinking soda in place of calcium-rich beverages.

- *Menstrual history.* An increased risk of osteoporosis is associated with delayed puberty in males or females, and **amenorrhea** in females (lack of menstrual periods for 3 months or more), whether related to an eating disorder, excessive exercise, or other causes. Women who are currently pregnant or breastfeeding usually have some transient bone loss, but this is reversed after the pregnancy and/or after breastfeeding is discontinued. Interestingly, women with more than 10 pregnancies appear to have the same risk of developing osteoporosis as women who have never been pregnant.

- *Menopause.* Menopause is the most significant factor when it comes to being at risk for osteoporosis. The loss of estrogen at menopause is the most common reason why women get osteoporosis. This drop in estrogen causes bone to be lost rapidly. Only 5% of postmenopausal women have osteoporosis from a source other than loss of estrogen.

- *Body weight and* **body mass index (BMI)**. Slender, small-boned women are at greater risk than overweight, large-boned women. BMI is a calculation that takes into account both weight and height; there are ranges established to identify underweight (<18), normal weight (18–25), overweight (>25), and obese (>30). If your BMI is low (<22), your

Amenorrhea

Absence of menstruation for 3 months or more.

Body mass index (BMI)

A calculation that takes into account both weight and height; there are ranges established to identify underweight (<18), normal weight (18–25), overweight (>25), and obese (>30). The calculation is weight (in pounds) divided by height (in inches) squared, and then multiply this number by 704.5.

risk for osteoporosis is increased, even though a BMI between 18 and 25 is considered normal. A BMI of 26–28 provides some protection, and a BMI of >28 increases risk because of the association with reduced activity. If you are > 5' 4" tall and weigh 127 pounds or less, or if your BMI is <22, you are more at risk for osteoporosis. You can calculate your BMI by taking your weight (in pounds), dividing it by your height (in inches) squared, and then multiplying this number by 704.5. If you don't want to do the math, you can have it calculated for you by visiting the Internet (*www.obesity.org*).

- *Poor nutrition.* Inadequate intake of calcium, vitamin D, citric acid, and phosphorus (or excessive intake of phosphorus) can cause weak bones with decreased bone mass. If you have a diet deficient in calcium, phosphorus, and Vitamin D, you are at increased risk of developing osteoporosis. A diet high in salt or excessively high in protein or fiber can also adversely affect bone because salt increases the excretion of calcium and excessive fiber, or protein can interfere with calcium consumption or absorption. Having a strict vegetarian diet (no foods that are animal-based) is associated with osteoporosis for two reasons: strict vegetarians avoid dairy products, an important source of calcium and vitamin D; and they also tend to have a lower BMI (around 20), which is also linked to osteoporosis.

- *Medications.* Some medications cause either an increase in bone loss or a decrease in bone formation. The following medications are some that increase your risk of osteoporosis: anticonvulsants, thyroid hormone, corticosteroids, lithium, methotrexate, gonadotropin-releasing hormone (GnRH), cholesteramine, heparin, warfarin, and antacids containing aluminum (see Question 15).

- *Medical conditions.* There are certain conditions that are associated with an increased risk of osteoporosis either because they interfere directly with bone development or indirectly due to medications required to treat them (see Question 16).
- **Sedentary lifestyle**. If you do not exercise, even if you have no other risk factors, you may still develop osteoporosis. Bones need the stress of exercise to keep bone formation equal to bone loss (see Questions 42–43).
- *Genetic factors.* Variations in or absence of a gene that regulates a specific protein receptor that is key to bone development may put you at risk for osteoporosis, sometimes a severe form of it. Several other genes controlling enzymes involved in bone development can affect your risk for osteoporosis.

Sedentary lifestyle
A way of living that involves little or no exercise.

Few studies have comprehensively evaluated specific risk factors for osteoporosis and osteoporosis-related fractures in men. The National Institutes of Health (NIH) is supporting the "Mr. O" Study of 5700 men who are 65 years of age and older to clarify the most important risks for men.

13. Can I change any of my risk factors?

You cannot change your age, gender, sex, race, fracture history, family history, menstrual history, time of menopause, genetic factors, and most medical conditions. You can, however, change some risk factors because most of them are related to lifestyle. Here's what you can do to lower your risk of developing osteoporosis or low bone mass:

- If you smoke, stop. If you don't already smoke, don't start. Appendix B lists resources for quitting smoking.

- If you drink alcohol, use moderation. More than two drinks per day increases your risk of osteoporosis as well as your risk of falling and breaking a bone.
- Replace caffeinated beverages with beverages rich in calcium. If you drink coffee or tea, consider adding milk. When drinking hot chocolate or cocoa, consider making it with milk to increase your calcium intake.
- Change your sedentary lifestyle to an active one by exercising daily (see Questions 42–44).
- Improve your diet. Take in adequate amounts of calcium, vitamin D, citric acid (found in citrus fruits), and phosphorus, and cut down on the amount of salt you eat. Be sure you get adequate amounts of protein and fiber, but remember that excessive amounts of fiber and protein can interfere with absorption of needed nutrients for bone development, unless you also supplement with calcium in your diet (see Questions 47–53).
- Ask your clinician if you could substitute medications that you are taking with ones that are less likely to cause bone loss or that will protect bones (see Question 15).
- If you have any medical conditions that put you at greater risk for bone loss, discuss with your clinician how your condition could be managed to reduce the risk of jeopardizing your bone health. For example, if you have an eating disorder, discuss getting the help you need to resume eating a healthy diet. Or if your BMI is less than 18 (meaning you are underweight), get the help you need to gain enough weight to have a healthier BMI. Although having a BMI of < 22 increases your risk for osteoporosis, exercising and maintaining a healthy BMI (18–25) is important for overall health. Exercise will also reduce your risk for osteoporosis.

- If you are exercising to the point of not having menstrual periods (amenorrhea), consider reducing the amount of time that you exercise or try taking in more calories to make up for the extra expenditure of calories from extreme exercise.
- If you are experiencing moderate to severe symptoms of postmenopause such as hot flashes and night sweats, talk with your clinician about taking estrogen to help relieve your symptoms as well as lower your risk of osteoporosis.

Grace's comment:

Well, being Black, I didn't really think it was a big problem for me. But my girlfriend just found out she has osteoporosis, and she has to take medication for it! She told me to get tested, so I talked to my doctor about it. He said we don't need to test for it until after my periods stop, that the estrogen I have in my body helps protect my bones, but that after the estrogen goes down due to menopause, then I will need to be tested. I asked what else I can do to protect my bones now and he said regular exercise, vitamins C and D, and calcium. And he said it is good that I don't smoke. So I learned that I can be at risk, too!

14. I have always worked hard to stay thin. Now that I have osteoporosis, I'm wondering if that was such a good idea. What's the connection between body weight and bones?

It really depends on how thin you are. Question 12 explains how to calculate your BMI. If your BMI is less than 22, then your weight is a risk factor for osteoporosis. You say that you have worked hard to stay thin.

Did you have to work hard in the sense that you were on a stringent diet and may not have had adequate intake of calcium, vitamin D, and protein? Or did you exercise excessively to stay thin? Both lifestyles could interfere with the normal process of bone breakdown and bone formation. If you had very low body weight as a child or adolescent, it's possible that you never reached peak bone mass.

Obesity

Condition of being severely overweight based on body mass index greater than 30, and associated with many health problems.

Obesity (BMI > 30) can also contribute to the development of osteoporosis, usually because people who are obese tend to be less active and, most importantly, they tend to exercise less. Lack of exercise is correlated directly with bone loss (see Question 42). But being overweight or obese is not all bad when it comes to bone health. The mere act of carrying around extra weight can increase the stress on bones, which contributes to the making of new bone. More muscle mass and higher **bone turnover** are also generally present in individuals who are overweight or obese. Both men and women who are overweight or obese have more circulating sex hormones, which assist in maintaining normal bone mass. Still, it's not clear if being overweight actually lowers the risk of fracture. Some older studies indicate that the risk of fracture is reduced in overweight women. But in later studies this risk is the same as those for normal-weight women. Unfortunately, being obese carries with it enormous health problems, so it's still considered advisable for overweight individuals to lose weight.

Bone turnover

The process of breaking down bone and forming new bone in its place, a process that occurs throughout life. When bone is growing (during childhood through early adulthood) new formation exceeds breakdown; later in life breakdown exceeds formation.

The bad news for you, as a very thin person, is that lower body weight (< 127 pounds or BMI < 22) is definitely linked to a higher risk of fracture. So, if you are thin and older, you are more likely to fracture your hip if you fall than your overweight counterparts, who may have denser bones and more fat to pad their falls.

And if you lose weight, intending to or not, your risk of hip fracture still goes up.

So, for you, being very thin, gaining enough weight to reach a BMI between 22 and 25 would be advisable after a discussion with your clinician. Reducing the potential for fracture should be your goal (see Questions 42–53 and 86).

15. Could I be taking any medications that affect bone health?

There are several types of medications that can put you at greater risk for developing osteopenia and osteoporosis. These types of medications are believed to decrease bone mass either by accelerating bone breakdown or by interfering with new bone formation. Some drugs may also interfere with the body's use of vitamin D and parathyroid hormone. However, certain medications cause bone loss and we just don't know why.

Glucocorticosteroids (prednisone, prednisolone, cortisone, glucocorticoids, steroids, adrenocorticotropic hormone [ACTH], Orapred®, Pediapred®, Prelone®) are the main group of medications associated with secondary osteoporosis. They cause more osteoporosis than any other medication. The glucocorticosteroids, also called corticosteroids or more commonly just steroids, can be taken orally, inhaled, injected, or used topically (through the skin) or intravenously. The oral, intravenous, and injected forms of steroids are the most damaging to bones. The long-term effects of inhaled or topical steroids on bone have not been well studied, so are not as well understood. Steroids are most often used in the treatment of asthma and other chronic lung diseases such as cystic fibrosis, emphysema, and sarcoidosis; rheumatologic disorders such as rheumatoid arthritis and lupus; skin diseases such as psoriasis and eczema; and inflammatory bowel diseases such as Crohn's and ulcerative colitis. Steroid (glucocorticoid) medications can cause osteoporosis for several reasons. First, they interfere with calcium absorption from food. Second, they may increase the amount of calcium lost through the kidneys. Third, they interfere directly with bone formation and with the production of testosterone and estrogen, which are hormones necessary for bone formation. And last, steroids can interfere with the ability to perform bone-strengthening exercises and increase fracture risk by causing muscle weakness and exercise intolerance.

Glucocorticoid-induced osteoporosis (GIO) can occur with as little as 3 months of treatment. If you are treated for longer than 6 months, you have a 50% chance of developing osteoporosis. And if you are treated long-term, you also have a 50% chance of sustaining a fracture related to osteoporosis. Doses at or above 5 mg per day are believed to stop new bone formation, causing rapid bone loss (see Question 88). Several medications used to treat osteoporosis and osteopenia carry an indication for use in patients taking long-term steroids at doses at or above 7.5 mg per day. Many clinicians will start therapy even if the steroid dose is 5 mg per day to slow or prevent additional bone loss (see Question 55).

The long-term use of the following medications also puts you at greater risk for osteoporosis:

- *Levothyroxine* (such as Synthroid®, Levathroid®, Unithyroid®, Levoxyl®, Eltroxin®) is used in the treatment of hypothyroidism (underactive thyroid gland).
- *Anticonvulsants* (such as Dilantin® [phenytoin]; phenobarbitol; Tegretol®, Carbatrol® [carbamazepine]; Depakote® [divalproex]; Depacon® [valproate]) are used in the treatment of seizure disorders.

- *Methotrexate* is used in the treatment of certain cancers and some chronic conditions such as rheumatoid arthritis and psoriasis.
- *Heparin®* and *Coumadin®* (warfarin) are used to prevent or dissolve blood clots resulting from immobility, pulmonary embolism, venous thrombosis, or atrial fibrillation.
- *Lithium* (Lithobid®, Eskalith®) is used in the treatment of manic depression (bipolar disorder), mania, and schizoaffective disorders.
- *Gonadotropin-releasing hormone agonists (GnRHa)* (such as Lupron or its generic equivalent, leuprolide acetate) are used to reduce estrogen levels in premenopausal women with endometriosis and fibroids; they are also used to reduce testosterone levels in men with prostate cancer. Because GnRHa reduces both estrogen and testosterone levels, it has a damaging effect on bone and is usually prescribed for only 3 to 6 months at a time. Bone density is closely monitored if it is used for longer periods.
- *Antacids containing aluminum* (such as Amphogel®, Maalox®, Mylanta®) are used in the treatment of indigestion. Some clinicians advise switching to a nonaluminum-containing antacid, such as Tums®, Di-Gel®, or Rolaids®, if you need to use antacids long-term. A list of antacids and their contents can be accessed through a Web site provided in Appendix B.
- *Medroxyprogesterone acetate injection* (Depo-Provera® contraceptive injection) is usually used as birth control in women. Recently, the FDA announced that it was mandating a label change to highlight the risk of bone loss with prolonged use (i.e., >2 years) of Depo-Provera. It is not clear if the loss is reversible when the every-3-months injections are stopped, but prior research with postmenopausal women indicated that previous use of Depo-Provera did not

have an effect on bone density after menopause, and more recent research with adolescent girls showed that bone density was preserved if they also took estrogen supplements while on the Depo-Provera.

- *Proton pump inhibitors* (Aciphex®, Nexium®, Prevacid®, Prilosec®, Prilosec OTC®, Protonix®, Zegerid®) are used to treat acid reflux and ulcers.
- *Selective seratonin reuptake inhibitors (SSRIs)* (such as Paxil®, Prozac®, Zoloft®, and others) are used to treat depression.
- *Thiazolidinedione (TZD)* (Actos®, Avandia®) is used to treat diabetes.

If you are taking or using any of these medications, you should have a discussion with your clinician about possible substitutes that would be equally as effective for treating your condition but would not jeopardize your bone health. You might also discuss having your bone health monitored and taking medications intended to treat and prevent further bone loss (see Questions 23–25, and 55).

You may also be taking medications that can actually improve your bone health. If you are taking estrogen either alone or in combination with a progestin for the treatment of menopausal symptoms, your bones will benefit and you can expect to have less bone loss (see Question 64).

If you are one of more than 8 million people taking statins (e.g., Mevacor®, Zocor®, Lipitor®) to lower your cholesterol, you may have the added benefit of improving your bone density and reducing your risk of fractures. Through an unknown mechanism, statins increase the levels of a bone-forming protein. Some studies have shown that statins can reduce the risk of hip fractures by as much as 30%. Other studies do not link statin use with a decreased risk of fracture and suggest that further study of the relationship between statins and bone health is needed. Although they may increase bone density, statins are not used to treat or prevent osteoporosis.

If you are taking a thiazide diuretic, such as Diuril®, Aquazide®, hydrochlorothiazide (HCTZ), and Esidrix®, to lower your blood pressure, you may be preventing bone loss, at least while you're taking it. Thiazide diuretics decrease the amount of calcium you lose through your kidneys and therefore increase the amount of calcium your body has available for bone formation. Although not prescribed for osteoporosis treatment or prevention, this class of medications also substantially cuts the risk of osteoporosis-related fractures. Once the medication is stopped, however, the benefits to bone health stop as well.

16. Are there any illnesses or medical conditions that are associated with osteoporosis?

If you have certain illnesses, you are definitely more at risk for developing osteoporosis either because of the illness itself or because the medications used to treat the underlying illness interfere with bone development (see Question 15).

Some illnesses, such as hyperthyroidism and Cushing's syndrome, increase the speed with which bone is broken down. Other illnesses, such as cystic fibrosis and celiac disease, interfere with bone formation by impeding the body's absorption or production of the nutrients needed for bone development. In fact, 3% to 4% of those with osteoporosis have **gluten intolerance**, the allergy to wheat that occurs in celiac disease. People with gluten intolerance cannot absorb the correct amount of calcium and vitamin D from their intestines. One of the problems

Gluten intolerance

Allergy to wheat, which occurs in celiac disease. Can cause intestinal absorption problems.

is that many people have minor symptoms and do not even know they have an allergy to wheat. Gluten intolerance can also occur later in life.

Table 1 lists illnesses and medical conditions that can interfere with good bone health. Most of the illnesses

Table 1   Medical Conditions That Cause or Increase Risk for Secondary Osteoporosis

Acromegaly	Adrenal Insufficiency	Alcoholism	Amyloidosis
Androgen Insensitivity	Ankylosing Spondolytis	Anorexia Nervosa	Athletic Amenorrhea
Breastfeeding	Calcium Deficiency	Celiac Disease	Cholestatic Liver Disease
Chronic Liver Disease	Chronic Obstructive Pulmonary Disease	Chronic Metabolic Acidosis	Congestive Heart Failure
Cushing's Syndrome	Cystic Fibrosis	Depression	Diabetes Mellitus, Type 1
Ehlers-Danlos Syndrome	Emphysema	End Stage Renal Disease	Epilepsy
Gastric Disease Operations (Gastrectomy/ Bypass)	Gaucher's Disease	Glycogen Storage Diseases	Hemochromatosis
Hemophelia	Homocystinuria	Hyperadrenocorticism	Hypercalciuria
Hyperpara-thyroidism	Hyperprolactinemia	Hypogonadism	Hypophosphatasia in Adults
Idiopathic Hypercalciuria	Idiopathic Scoliosis	Immobilization	Inflammatory Bowel Disease
Klinefelter's Syndrome	Leukemias	Lupus	Mastocytosis
Malabsorption Syndromes	Malnutrition	Marfan Syndrome	Menkes Kinky Hair Syndrome

(cont.)

Table 1   Medical Conditions That Cause or Increase Risk for Secondary Osteoporosis (*cont.*)

Multiple Sclerosis	Muscular Dystrophy	Myeloma and Some Cancers	Organ Transplantation
Osteogenesis Imperfecta	Panhypopituitarism	Porphyria	Posttransplant Bone Disease
Pregnancy	Premature Ovarian Failure	Primary Biliary Cirrhosis	Renal Tubular Acidosis
Rheumatoid Arthritis	Riley-Day Syndrome	Sarcoidosis	Sickle Cell Disease
Thalassemia	Thyrotoxicosis	Turner's Syndrome	Vitamin D Deficiency

Sources: U.S. Department of Health and Human Services. *Bone Health and Osteoporosis: A Report of the Surgeon General.* Rockville, MD: U.S. Department of Health and Human Services, Office of the Surgeon General; 2004.
and
Dawson-Hughes B, Lindsay R, Khosla S, et al. *Clinician's Guide to Prevention and Treatment of Osteoporosis.* Washington DC: National Osteoporosis Foundation; 2008; available at: http://www.nof.org/professionals/clinicians_Guide.htm accessed September 29, 2009.

listed are chronic; however, other illnesses or conditions can be shorter term, meaning that the bone loss caused by the illness or condition can be reversible. For example, pregnancy and lactation cause temporary bone loss because calcium is needed by the developing fetus and the infant who is breastfeeding. But pregnancy- and lactation-associated bone loss stops either after delivery of the baby or the weaning of the baby from the breast. Interestingly, this transient bone loss does not have long-term effects and is not changed by taking additional calcium during pregnancy or lactation. **Hypogonadism,** or low testosterone levels, is a chronic condition that affects men and can interfere with normal bone development.

Individuals with chronic kidney disease usually have high levels of phosphorus in the blood. High blood levels of phosphorus put them at increased risk for osteoporosis. They must take a special medication

Hypogonadism

Inadequate testicular or ovarian function most commonly causing low levels of testosterone.

called Renagel (sevelamer) that binds the extra phosphorus and allows the body to excrete the surplus through the intestines. Those who are on **dialysis** often have their blood checked weekly for phosphorus levels and their Renagel dosage adjusted accordingly.

Because depression is definitely a medical condition associated with low bone mass and decreased bone mineral density (BMD), some clinicians recommend screening for osteoporosis in older individuals with major depression who may not have other risk factors. Depression is also associated with an increased risk for falls. It is not entirely clear whether the diagnosis and effects of having osteoporosis cause the depression or if the chemical imbalance or sedentary lifestyle resulting from depression interferes with bone development.

There are several reasons why asthma also can be a serious risk factor for developing osteoporosis. First, steroid medications are often used to decrease inflammation of the airway. These medications are known to increase bone loss (see Question 15). Second, many asthma sufferers are convinced that milk and milk products increase mucus production, and they therefore avoid a group of foods that contain calcium. They may also avoid milk because they believe it will trigger an asthma attack, but unless you are allergic to milk, there is no evidence that this will occur. And last, exercise can be a trigger for an asthmatic attack. Those who suffer from exercise-induced asthma may become sedentary, avoiding the weight-bearing or resistive exercises required for bone growth.

Marianne's comment:

I have been on hemodialysis for kidney disease for well over a year. I have to be very careful about eating foods

Dialysis

Process by which impurities and toxic substances are removed from the body either by filtering blood through a machine or infusing fluids into the abdominal cavity that remove wastes; required for those who do not have adequately functioning kidneys.

that are too high in phosphorus because my kidneys are not able to process the phosphorus correctly. My nephrologist does not want my phosphorus levels to get too high because calcium will be taken from my bones, making them weaker. Also, the phosphorus makes my skin itch. Although I take Renagel to keep the phosphorus levels down, the dialysis also removes phosphorus from my blood. Food labels don't contain phosphorus levels, so it's sometimes difficult to know how much phosphorus I'm getting. I have to make different food choices than I would normally like to make! For example, I should choose a Popsicle instead of ice cream, a bagel instead of biscuits, and gelatin instead of pudding. I have to be careful of sodium and potassium as well. I also take 1500 mg of calcium with vitamin D every day, and so far, my annual bone density tests have not shown any osteoporosis, even though I know that having kidney disease can weaken my bones.

17. How will I know if I have osteoporosis? Are there any signs or symptoms?

Because osteoporosis and osteopenia are not painful conditions, you will not know that you have either one unless you break a bone or you have **bone mineral density testing**.

Naturally, if you suspect you have broken a bone, get medical help immediately. But in the following situations, you may be uncertain, so it is still wise to call your clinician:

- Pain and bruising following a fall that occurred without a lot of force or trauma could indicate that you have broken a bone. Don't say to yourself,

Bone mineral density (BMD) tests
Safe, painless, and noninvasive tests to evaluate bone mineral density.

"It was only a little fall—I couldn't have broken a bone." While not common, it is important to discuss such injuries with your clinician.

- Back pain that comes on suddenly in the spine can mean that you have one or more **vertebral fractures** resulting from osteoporosis. This is different from the back pain associated with a muscle spasm. Even if you have just bent forward to reach for something or slipped in the bathtub, you can still get a fracture in your spine if you have osteoporosis.

One physical sign indicating that you have osteoporosis is loss of height. So, if you shrink in height as measured in your annual physical exam, you should ask to be screened for osteoporosis, particularly if your clinician doesn't notice or doesn't recommend screening.

Vertebral fracture

A fracture of the body of a vertebra (spine bone) that collapses it and makes it thinner and weaker. Usually results from osteoporosis but can also result from complications of cancer or some injuries.

18. If osteoporosis doesn't hurt, what impact does it have on my health?

Osteoporosis can affect your health in many ways, directly and indirectly:

- You become much more susceptible to fractures. Fractures, depending on which bone you break, can cause physical immobility and impairment of your general health, as well as financial problems and social isolation. Fractures can lead to death. If you are 50 or older with osteoporosis, you have a 1 in 2 chance of having an osteoporosis-related fracture during the remainder of your lifetime.
- Vertebral fractures caused by osteoporosis can severely affect the quality of your life in many areas,

such as social functioning, overall health, emotional health, bodily pain, and vitality. The acute back pain associated with vertebral fractures and the healing process can be very debilitating. Being unable to do activities of daily living without pain can cause you to stop moving physically and mentally: physically because of pain or physical impairment, and mentally because of fears of further injury and resulting isolation and possibly depression. Pain associated with fractures in other bones can cause similar scenarios with fear, frustration, and reluctance to do the activities to which you've become accustomed. There are many hazards to being immobile, all of them affecting your health in a negative way (see Question 83).

- Getting shorter and, in some cases, developing a deformity of your back can cause problems physically and emotionally. A deformity called **kyphosis** (sometimes called "**dowager's hump**") develops when the front edges of the bones of the spine collapse due to osteoporosis and tiny fractures. **Figure 6** depicts the changes in your spine resulting from osteoporosis. The deformed spine does not just make you shorter; it can compress organs in your chest and abdomen, making it difficult for you to breathe and digest food appropriately (see Question 84). Men and women with this disfigurement can have poor body image or low self-esteem, sometimes causing them to withdraw from social activities. Even finding clothes that fit well and look right can be difficult, further contributing to social isolation and depression.

- Depression can be a direct result of osteoporosis, fractures, the fear of falling, and the resulting social isolation. You may become depressed because you are isolated from friends and family as a result, for

Kyphosis

A type of physical deformity that develops when the front edges of the bones of the spine collapse because of osteoporosis and tiny fractures. Also called dowager's hump.

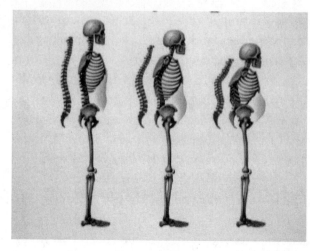

Figure 6   Progression of spine deformity and the loss of height. Note that organs become compressed or shifted in position with progression of osteoporosis. Courtesy of the National Association of Nurse Practitioners in Women's Health (NPWH).

example, of a hip fracture. Later, when your hip has healed, you might become fearful of venturing out again, causing you ongoing isolation from friends and family (see Question 82).

• Over 65,000 women die from hip fractures every year. But if you survive, chances are you will be disabled. Just one hip fracture that results from osteoporosis can give you lasting disability. Twenty percent of women with fractures will never leave a nursing home. Another 50% will be permanently incapacitated.

• Your overall health can suffer when you have osteoporosis. You may be malnourished from not getting enough of the nutrients that keep your bones healthy. As a result of fractures, you may become less physically active, causing further weakening of your bones and muscles. This loss of strength can cause rapid deterioration in your overall health.

19. When should I be tested for osteoporosis? Will my tests be covered by insurance?

The National Osteoporosis Foundation recommends bone mineral density (BMD) testing on the following individuals:

- If you are a woman aged 65 or older or a man aged 70 or older, you should be tested for osteoporosis even if you have no other risk factors.
- If you are a postmenopausal woman under age 65 or a man aged 50 to 70, and you have clinical risk factors that put you at risk for bone loss or fractures, you should be tested. Generally, risk factors include the following (also see Questions 12 and 13):

    Fractures in adulthood (especially after age 50)

    Low-trauma fractures

    Family history of osteoporosis

    Genetic factors

    Sedentary lifestyle

    Nutritional deficiencies

    Excessive alcohol, soda, or caffeine intake

    Cigarette smoking

    Low body weight or body mass index (BMI) below 22

    Certain medications (especially steroids; see Question 15)

    Low testosterone levels in men

    Amenorrhea (no menstrual periods) from excessive exercise

    Hormonal imbalances (prior to menopause)

    Anorexia nervosa

    Certain medical conditions (see Question 16)

- If you are a postmenopausal woman and have recently stopped taking estrogen, you should be tested.
- If you are a woman experiencing the menopause transition and have specific risk factors that are associated with a higher risk for fracture, such as low weight, use of a high-risk medication, or previous low-trauma fracture, you should be tested.
- If you are a man or a woman who had a fracture when you were over age 50, you should be tested.
- If you are a woman or a man with a medical condition (e.g., arthritis) or are taking a medication (e.g., corticosteroid at 5 mg or more per day for 3 months or more) that is associated with bone loss or low bone mass, you should be tested.
- If you are considering taking medication for osteoporosis, you should be tested.
- If you are being treated for osteoporosis, you should be tested to monitor how well the treatment is working.
- If knowing that you have bone loss would prompt you to use therapy, you should be tested.

You will note that several of the above recommendations refer specifically to men. Male patients and their clinicians should discuss their risk factors for osteoporosis, just as women should. Screening for bone loss is important for both women and men. Insurance coverage for testing of both men and women varies by insurance company. However, Medicare does cover bone density testing for those 65 or older who:

- Have vertebral abnormalities (e.g., a hump or severe curvature)
- Are estrogen-deficient (postmenopausal) women with a clinical risk for osteoporosis
- Take or plan to take long-term glucocorticoid therapy (5 mg or more per day for 3 or more months)

- Have primary hyperparathyroidism (overproduction of parathyroid hormone interferes with bone development)
- Are being monitored for effects of or response to approved osteoporosis treatments (see Part 3)

Testing may be repeated every 2 years, if you have Medicare. If you have medical coverage other than Medicare, you should check the guidelines for retesting with your insurance company.

Mark's comment:

I had ulcerative colitis for many years, and I was treated with steroids to control the diarrhea and bleeding. My nurse practitioner always talked to me about exercise, calcium, and vitamin D to make sure I protected my bones as much as possible. She also sent me for a bone density test. The people at the testing place were surprised—they said she was really paying attention and that it was unusual but really good that she sent me to get tested. They said bone loss happens too often to guys like me, but that most clinicians don't think to test for it. I guess I am one of the lucky ones because my bones were OK—but my nurse practitioner still tested me every few years and made sure I was getting enough calcium. Now I don't take steroids anymore at all—I had surgery and they removed the part of the colon that caused my problems. I am so glad it is better, and that my bones are OK. I feel like I have my life ahead of me. I'm only 48, so keeping my bones strong now is really important.

20. If my clinician does not discuss screening for osteoporosis, at what age should I make sure that I am screened?

You and your clinician should discuss your bone health during every annual exam, regardless of your age. Your calcium and vitamin D intake, your level of physical activity, and your lifestyle factors such as smoking and drinking alcohol can affect bone health at any age.

If you believe that you have one or more risk factors for developing osteoporosis, it is important to discuss being screened with your clinician (see Question 12). The Surgeon General, in his 2004 report on bone health, advises that the following "red flags" at any age should warrant further assessment for osteoporosis or other bone diseases:

- Fracture following mild or moderate trauma (e.g., fracture after falling from standing height or less; see Question 74)
- Low body weight or weight loss of over 1% per year in elders
- Loss of height or progressive curvature of the spine
- Family member with bone disease
- Delayed puberty
- Atypical ending of menstrual periods (e.g., early menopause)
- High levels of alkaline phosphatase (a liver enzyme) or serum calcium in persons who are otherwise healthy
- Anorexia nervosa
- Amenorrhea, either due to intense physical activity, eating disorders, or hormonal imbalances
- Treatment with medications that affect bone remodeling (e.g., glucocorticosteroids; see Question 15)
- Presence of disease that is associated with secondary osteoporosis (see Question 16)
- Overproduction of thyroid or parathyroid hormones or intake of high thyroid hormone doses
- Prolonged immobilization

- Calcium deficiency (caused by inadequate calcium intake or poor absorption)
- Vitamin D deficiency (caused by low intake through diet or **supplements** or by poor absorption)

21. Can my clinician tell if I have osteoporosis during my annual check-up?

It is very important that your clinician take a good history during your annual check-up. The history is particularly important because osteoporosis is not painful unless you break a bone. Your clinician should ask you about the following:

- Family history of osteoporosis
- Personal history of fractures
- Presence of chronic or new acute back pain
- Menstrual history including menopause (surgical or natural); amenorrhea
- Medications that can cause secondary osteoporosis (see Question 15)
- History of illnesses that are associated with secondary osteoporosis (see Question 16)
- Lifestyle factors such as cigarette smoking, heavy alcohol consumption, and activity level
- Intake of calcium and vitamin D

After taking a thorough history, your clinician will examine you. For the purposes of detecting osteoporosis or for conditions that put you at increased risk of developing osteoporosis, your clinician should pay particular attention to the following:

- Height loss—actually measuring your height using a stadiometer is important
- Low body weight on petite frame, BMI < 22; or BMI > 28

Supplements

Additional doses of vitamins, minerals, or other dietary substances; usually taken to enhance diet to get the recommended amount for your age, gender, and medical conditions.

Risk Factors and Testing

- Elevated pulse and blood pressure (for overproduction of thyroid hormone)
- Tooth loss
- Enlarged thyroid gland
- Tenderness over bones of your back
- Curvature of the spine (kyphosis)
- Limited range of motion in the spine, shoulders, elbows, wrists, hips, knees, or ankles
- Shortened distance from the rib cage to the front edge of the pelvis while lying down face-up (happens when spine begins to curve from repeated fractures)
- In men—smaller testicles may indicate loss of testosterone (related to hypogonadism)
- In women—breast and pelvic exams may show evidence of estrogen loss.

Even after collecting all of this information, your clinician cannot determine if you have osteoporosis. They use this information to determine your risk for osteoporosis and then will order testing if needed (see Question 23).

Penny's comment:

Since age 65, I have had a complete yearly physical, blood work, urinalysis, and so forth. When I reached age 79, my doctor thought it would be a good idea to have a bone density test. My left hip showed the beginnings of bone loss, but only to the degree of "osteopenia." I then started taking 1200 milligrams of calcium, plus vitamin D.

At this year's exam, my doctor noted it had been 3 years since my last bone density test. I was sent to a bone specialist's office for the tests. I had a scan of my ulna and radius. After that I was led into another room for a spinal x-ray because I had a compression fracture a little more than a year ago in the thoracic region of the spine. My hip was also tested.

Lying on that white x-ray table was an ordeal I would not like to face again. Not only was the room cold, but also the hard smooth surface of the table was like ice, and maneuvering me into the position they desired was very painful. I do have the beginnings as well of arthritis, and some of the movement, not noticeable on standing and normal movement, caused a great amount of discomfort.

After the tests were done and the results printed out, I was given a stack of papers to look at, and they were compared against the bone structures of some unknown 30-year-old to give me a score that assured me of the diagnosis. After all the tests, I was diagnosed with the real thing—osteoporosis.

It was a shock to me. Two years ago, my orthopedic doctor told me at the time I was put in the brace for the compression fracture in my back that this might happen again and to keep the brace handy. He also mentioned that there were some signs of arthritis at the time. But he never actually told me that I had osteoporosis.

When you reach age 82 plus, you expect some aches and pains and creaking joints and a feeling of malaise once in a while, but you never put a name to it because the next day it can be better.

Now that I have been told unequivocally that I have osteoporosis, I feel mentally stooped inside. From what I can tell by looking in the mirror, though, my spine is not nearly as curved as those on the diagrams hanging on all four walls in the osteoporosis specialist's office.

I was told I had a choice of three medications to keep the deterioration of the bone to a minimum. I chose weekly Actonel®. I have to be cautious and take it exactly as directed so that I don't get more stomach upset than I already have.

I was also told to take an extra 400 mg of vitamin D once a day to ensure a better response to the 1200 mg of calcium I am also taking. The calcium levels in my blood are normal. The specialist also wanted me to exercise. I told her that lifting art supplies for my painting class, walking up and down the aisles of the grocery store every day, and doing my leg exercises at home would have to be enough exercise.

I can laugh, and groan, and complain about how growing old takes courage. I just hope that between now and the time I return to the doctor, I will have regained my sense of humor, and be grateful the sun is still shining and that I am NOT walking with a cane, a walker, or sitting slumped in a wheelchair.

22. My clinician is concerned about my loss of height of 1 inch in the past year. Does that mean I definitely have osteoporosis?

Once you reach midlife, you should be measured for height each year that you go for an annual check-up. In addition to height, your spine should be assessed for kyphosis (prominent upper curve of the spine giving a hunched-over appearance). Although loss of height can mean other things such as poor posture, decreased muscle strength, or even poor measuring techniques, it can be a good indicator of bone loss in the spine. In fact, in one study, 75% of new vertebral fractures were found in individuals who had lost 1 to 2 inches in height.

Tiny compression fractures of the vertebrae can happen silently (without pain), reducing your height and causing the spine to curve. Figure 6 (Question 18) shows the progression from a normal spine to the curved spine, causing a loss of height. Your clinician is right to be concerned, and you should be further evaluated for osteoporosis.

23. How is osteoporosis diagnosed?

Conventional x-rays are not used to diagnose osteoporosis; however, osteoporosis can sometimes be seen on x-rays. The x-rays used to diagnose a fracture can show osteoporosis, but only if you have a significant amount of bone loss—that is, 30% to 40%.

There are, however, other tests that can be used specifically to evaluate your bone health. All bone mineral density (BMD) tests are safe, painless, and noninvasive. Most of the tests subject you to no more radiation than that received from the atmosphere during a cross-country airplane trip. One of the BMD tests uses ultrasound technology.

You should not be tested for bone density if you are pregnant or have had other x-ray studies that require dye within 2 weeks of bone density testing. Testing is limited for individuals who weigh more than 250 pounds. This is both because many machines can only hold individuals who weigh 250 pounds or less and because the more soft tissue there is, the harder it is to distinguish it from bone, making it difficult to obtain accurate results.

The "gold standard" (best test) for diagnosing osteoporosis or identifying osteopenia is **dual-energy x-ray absorptiometry (DXA)**. Because your hip, spine, or whole body may be evaluated using DXA, you will need to lie down on an x-ray type of table while a

Dual-energy x-ray absorptiometry (DXA)

A type of radiological test used to precisely determine bone mineral density with very little radiation.

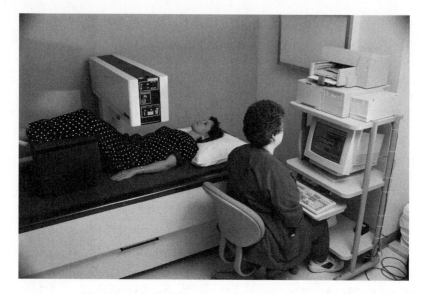

Figure 7　A woman getting a bone mineral density test with a DXA machine. The test is safe, noninvasive, and painless. © Photodisc.

Osteoarthritis

Inflammation and stiffness of the joints that usually occurs in older persons as a result of deterioration of the cartilage around the joints.

Peripheral dual-energy x-ray absorptiometry (pDXA)

A scan using the same technology as the DXA but measures bone density in the wrist, forearm, finger, or heel; it is only used for screening purposes, as a diagnosis of osteoporosis must be made with a DXA.

machine takes measurements of your bone density. The measurements and images of your bones are sent to a computer nearby, usually in the same room. **Figure 7** shows a woman undergoing bone mineral density testing with a DXA machine.

DXA scan measurements are very precise and use very little radiation. They are also the best tests for monitoring changes in bone density and evaluating effectiveness of treatments over time. It is best to have your bone density measured on the same machine and by the same technician each time you have it done, if possible. The presence of fractures, **osteoarthritis**, and calcifications (calcium deposits) can interfere with the accuracy of BMD testing, particularly of the spine (see Questions 31–32).

The **peripheral dual-energy x-ray absorptiometry (pDXA)** scan uses the same technology as the DXA but measures bone density in your wrist, forearm, finger, or heel (see Questions 24–25).

If a central DXA test shows osteoporosis at one or more sites, your clinician will most likely do some laboratory tests prior to confirming the diagnosis because your clinical history and laboratory results are needed before deciding if it is osteoporosis alone, or if there is another problem causing secondary osteoporosis or medication(s) causing bone loss (see Questions 9, 15, 16, and 33).

24. What is the difference between a DXA and a pDXA?

The DXA (or sometimes called the DEXA) and pDXA (or sometimes called pDEXA) are both used to evaluate bone density. The DXA takes up to 10 minutes to complete and the pDXA takes less than 5 minutes. The DXA measures bone density in the lumbar spine, the hip (also called proximal femur), the forearm, or the total body. The pDXA testing is usually done on the forearm at the wrist or on the heel of the foot, but it can also be used higher on the forearm or on the fingers. The pDXA machine is portable and can be used to screen bone density in large numbers of people, especially in rural areas and at health fairs. The DXA machines are not mobile and are far more expensive than the pDXA machines. DXA testing is done with the patient lying down and pDXA can be done with the patient sitting up. The DXA uses a very small amount of radiation and the pDXA even less.

The pDXA testing is only done for screening purposes. A diagnosis of osteoporosis can only be made using DXA. So if your pDXA shows some bone loss, your clinician would likely recommend a DXA to evaluate your hip and spine. pDXA testing is not considered appropriate for monitoring bone density in patients undergoing treatments for osteoporosis because response to treatments is not as evident in the bones of your hands, arms, and feet. pDXA testing on your forearm, usually your nondominant arm (for example, your left forearm if you are right handed), is not recommended if your forearm has been previously fractured, if it has a dialysis graft site, if it has been subject to prolonged immobilization, or if there is severe weakness or paralysis of that arm.

25. Are there other tests that are used to diagnose osteoporosis?

While other tests can be used to diagnose osteoporosis, the WHO has established the guidelines for diagnosis based only on the results of DXA testing. So most other methods for identifying osteoporosis or osteopenia are used for screening, and then if the screening test suggests reduced bone density, a DXA is ordered to make a diagnosis. The following are the other tests that are available but less widely used:

Single energy x-ray absorptiometry (SXA)
Type of radiograph where the bone mineral density test is done on the wrist or heel while the body part is submerged in water.

Quantitative computed tomography (QCT)
Type of radiography that uses CT scan technology to measure the bone density in the spine.

- **Single energy x-ray absorptiometry (SXA)**, like the pDXA, is done at the wrist or the heel. Interestingly, the body part being measured for bone density is submerged in a water bath.
- **Quantitative computed tomography (QCT)** is a method of testing that uses CT scan technology to measure bone density in the spine. Although it provides accurate measurements, the major drawback to this test is that it exposes the patient to 50 times more radiation than the DXA test. QCT is more

expensive than DXA and takes between 10 and 20 minutes to perform. It is a good option for people who have arthritis in the spine because the QCT results are not affected by changes due to arthritis that can interfere with DXA results.

- **Peripheral quantitative computed tomography (pQCT)** uses the same technology as the QCT but measures bone density in the forearm or wrist. This test is not routinely ordered and is used primarily in the research field.
- **Radiographic absorptiometry (RA)** is actually a conventional x-ray used to measure bone density in the hand (primarily the middle bones of the 2nd, 3rd, and 4th fingers). Special software and scanning equipment can measure bone density. Radiation from this test is minimal.
- **Quantitative ultrasound (QUS)**, like other ultrasound techniques, uses sound waves instead of radiation. The heel, wrist, tibia bone in the leg, and a finger can be imaged and evaluated for bone mass.
- **Radiogrammetry** is a test that, like RA, uses conventional x-rays. Instead of fingers, however, two hand bones (metacarpals) are used to measure and compare bone density.

Figure 8 shows the tests that are used to measure bone density in various parts of the skeleton.

In addition to BMD tests, there are also **biochemical "markers"** that are measured in blood and urine to determine if specific therapies for osteoporosis are working. Biochemical marker measurements are not used for the purpose of diagnosing osteoporosis but sometimes for monitoring the progress of treatments (see Questions 39 and 69).

Risk Factors and Testing

Peripheral quantitative computed tomography (pQCT)

Type of radiography that uses the same technology as the QCT but measures bone density in the forearm or wrist; primarily used in research.

Radiographic absorptiometry (RA)

Conventional x-ray with software and scanning equipment used to measure bone density of the middle bones of the hand.

Quantitative ultrasound (QUS)

A type of radiological scan that uses sound waves to image the heel, wrist, tibia bone in the leg, and a finger for bone mass.

Radiogrammetry

A type of radiological test that, like RA, uses conventional x-rays; two hand bones (metacarpals) are used to measure and compare bone density.

Biochemical marker

Substance found in blood and urine that can be tested to determine the rate of bone turnover.

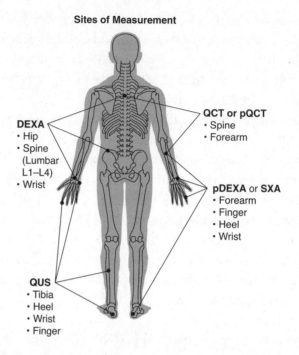

Figure 8   Sites in the body measured by different BMD tests. Courtesy of the National Association of Nurse Practitioners in Women's Health (NPWH).

26. How do I know which type of test should be ordered?

Tests for osteoporosis are either done to screen an individual to detect the presence of bone loss or done to monitor the progress of previously diagnosed bone loss. You may recall from Question 23 that the only tests used to diagnose osteoporosis are those that test the bone density of your spine or hip. Tests that are performed on **peripheral limbs** (hands, forearms, wrists, lower leg, and feet) are primarily used for screening. However, if you are obese, **peripheral bone mineral density testing** at the forearm is often used for diagnosis because most DXA machines are inaccurate for and cannot accommodate individuals who weigh more than 250 pounds.

The test that your clinician orders for you may be determined by many factors. Some of them are the availability of test sites and machines; your private insurance coverage or Medicare; and your individual medical situation, which includes your medical history, your risk factors for bone loss, whether you already have bone loss, and if you can travel to the specific testing site.

If you attend a health fair where you are screened for bone loss using a portable machine, there is not likely to be a choice of tests. And if the portable testing shows bone loss, your clinician may advise you to get a test of your spine or hip (DXA or QCT) to confirm a diagnosis of osteoporosis.

If you are reluctant to have a QCT due to the radiation or the expense, you should ask if there is an alternative test that could be done.

27. What if I live in a rural area and I can't get to a place with a DXA machine? Are there further tests that I would need?

DXA machines are the most widely available of all machines used for testing bone mineral density. However, some areas of the United States do not have access to DXA machines. Because it is important to have your bone density evaluated, particularly if you have risk factors for osteoporosis, you should still be evaluated using one of the screening tests that may be available in your area.

While it is preferable to have a test of your spine or hip to confirm a diagnosis of osteoporosis or determine if you have osteopenia, your clinician can still recommend preventive options and counsel you about nutrition and exercise for improving your bone health (see Part 3).

If you do not have access to any bone mineral density testing, it is still important to adhere to a regimen of **weight-bearing exercises** as well as a diet with sufficient calcium, vitamin D, and other nutrients to maintain healthy bones. You should also make every effort to prevent falls (see Question 79).

Weight-bearing exercise

Type of activity that places weight on certain bones; necessary for bone growth; examples are walking, dancing, and stair-climbing.

28. If I'm x-rayed for a broken bone, will osteoporosis, if I have it, show up on the x-ray? If it shows up on the x-ray, would I need further testing?

It usually takes about a 30% to 40% bone loss for osteoporosis to show up on conventional x-rays.

If you have advanced osteoporosis with significant bone loss, your x-rays may show osteoporosis. It usually takes about a 30% to 40% bone loss for osteoporosis to appear on conventional x-rays. Although x-rays are not used to diagnose osteoporosis, vertebral fractures are sometimes noted on conventional x-rays of the spine. If you have a chest x-ray, for example for pneumonia, vertebral fractures might be found incidentally, meaning that you may not have complained about them but they are nonetheless present and seen on the chest x-ray. Vertebral fractures noted on any type of x-ray are usually an indication that you have some degree of bone loss; however, further testing is still required after the fracture heals.

The fact that you have fractured a bone, particularly if it was due to a small amount of force or from a standing height or less, is more important in considering whether you need further testing for osteoporosis (see Question 74). It is important to establish a baseline of bone mass so that future therapies and treatments can be monitored for their effectiveness.

Any individual who has a vertebral (a bone in the spine) fracture or hip fracture is at high risk for osteoporosis, and while the fracture should be healed first (because fractures can sometimes interfere with the accuracy of DXA testing), further bone mineral density testing is still necessary. In case you are treated for any fracture through an emergency department or through a specialist, you should always update your primary care clinician about your fracture so that further testing can take place if necessary.

29. I've heard that x-rays of my teeth can be an indicator for osteoporosis. Is that true?

It is important to keep up with your oral health checkups throughout your entire life. When you go to the dentist, you may find out more than the condition of your teeth and gums—you may find out that you should be tested for osteoporosis. Although osteoporosis cannot be diagnosed from conventional bite-wing dental x-rays, periodontal (gum, tissues, and bone supporting teeth) disease can suggest that you have osteoporosis. Loss of teeth and bone loss in your jawbone can also indicate that you may have osteoporosis. Bone loss, depending on its extent, is sometimes visible on oral **panoramic x-rays**.

If you already have osteoporosis, your gum disease may become more severe. It is not clear yet whether low bone mass causes more rapid gum loss or if the inflammation of the gum tissue leads to more loss of bone density. Either way, if you have **periodontal disease**, you should discuss BMD testing with your clinician.

Panoramic x-rays

A type of radiography, usually of teeth and surrounding bones, such as the jawbone.

Periodontal disease

Disease of the gums, tissues, and bone supporting teeth.

As your gums become inflamed and recede, you may lose teeth. Tooth loss is definitely a predictor of osteoporosis. If an x-ray (usually a panoramic x-ray) of your jawbone shows bone loss, you are likely to have loss of bone mass in other bones as well.

Calcium and vitamin D intake is important not just for your bones but also for your teeth. So if you are not getting enough of either one, you are not only at risk for osteoporosis but also for tooth loss. If you have poor oral health, this does not mean that you definitely have weak bones. And on the other hand, if you have osteoporosis or osteopenia, it does not mean that you have bad teeth and gums.

Your oral health can offer clues that might prompt a discussion with your primary care clinician about osteoporosis.

Because osteoporosis is such a silent disease initially, it is important to consider every clue that you might have it. So, go to your dental professional twice a year for a cleaning and evaluation—your oral health can offer clues that might prompt a discussion with your primary care clinician about osteoporosis. And if you are contemplating tooth implants, it is critical to inform your dental professional if you have osteoporosis because tooth implants must be rooted in strong bone.

30. What should I do to prepare for the BMD tests? When my clinician orders the tests, how soon should they be done? If my provider can't schedule my tests for 6 weeks after they're ordered, is that OK?

Although many tables have a pad, some women are uncomfortable lying down on hard x-ray–type tables for BMD tests that measure the bone density of their hips or spine. You can ask for a pad or a wedge for under your knees if you are uncomfortable lying on the table. All BMD tests are essentially painless and noninvasive. There are no dyes to drink, no intravenous lines to be inserted. You don't need to fast for 2 days or go without eating and drinking after midnight. You should not, however, have BMD tests done if you have had studies with **contrast dye** within the past 2 weeks. You also should not have BMD testing while you are pregnant. You won't be able to undergo some of the BMD tests if you weigh over 250 pounds.

Do not take your calcium supplements for 24 hours before your test. Although the tests don't take long, wear comfortable clothing like sweatpants and a t-shirt. You should not wear clothes with metal clasps or metal zippers. Leave your underwire bra and bellybutton ring at home as well.

BMD testing is rarely ordered on an emergency basis. So, waiting a month or 6 weeks to get an appointment is okay. Naturally, when the tests are ordered, it's best to get them done as soon as you reasonably can.

31. My test results were reported as a T-score to my clinician. What is a T-score?

The results of your BMD tests will most likely be expressed as a **T-score**, which uses a mathematical formula and assigns your bone density results either a positive or negative number. Normally, density would be expressed as weight per volume, but because the bone images are only two dimensional, area must be used to calculate your results (grams per centimeter squared

Contrast dye

A dye that is given orally or intravenously for the purposes of focusing certain types of imaging tests; should not be taken within 2 weeks before having a bone mineral density test.

T-score

A positive or negative number denoting bone density in comparison with that of healthy young adults.

[g/cm^2]). Because there are different types of machines for BMD testing, a standard way of expressing the bone density measurements was developed. This method uses a formula comparing your individual results of BMD testing with the mean (average) bone density of healthy young adults of your same sex. The formula is expressed in **standard deviations** and looks like this:

$$\frac{\text{Patient's BMD} - \text{Young normal mean BMD}}{\text{Standard deviation of young normal mean}}$$

The WHO came up with the following classification of BMD testing results:

- T-score above −1.0 indicates that your bone mass is *normal* for your age.
- T-score between −1.0 and −2.5 indicates that you have *osteopenia (low bone mass)*.
- T-score −2.5 or lower indicates that you have *osteoporosis*.
- T-score −2.5 or lower plus the presence of one or more fragility fractures indicates that you have *severe osteoporosis*. A **fragility fracture** is a fracture of a bone that happens with little or no force or trauma, such as falling from your standing height or less (see Question 74).

In 1994, when the WHO developed this method of classification of results, the researchers felt it was important to present results in a way that related them to the lifetime risk of fracture. After all, understanding your risk for breaking bones is a major reason for doing the BMD testing. Bone density is about 10% to 12% lower for each standard deviation below normal (or BMD of 0). Likewise, the risk for fracture doubles

Standard deviation

A mathematical measure that indicates how far or how near something is to the mean (average).

Fragility fracture

Term used to describe a fracture that occurs with very little trauma or force and from a height that is usually not great enough to cause broken bones, usually indicating that the bone is weak. Also called an osteoporotic fracture.

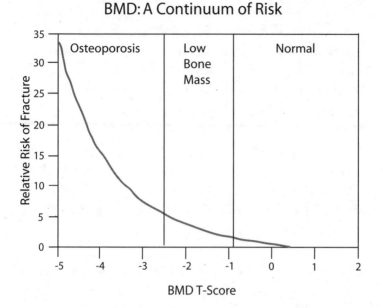

BMD: A Continuum of Risk

Figure 9   As the T-score decreases, the risk for fracture increases. Courtesy of the National Association of Nurse Practitioners in Women's Health (NPWH).

Source: Meunier PG et al. Clin Ther 1999;21:1025–1044.

with each standard deviation below normal bone density. So if your T-score is −1.0, your risk of having a fracture is roughly twice that of a young adult. If your T-score is −2.0, your risk is about 4 times higher, and if your T-score is −3.0, your risk for fracture is about 8 times higher than that of a young adult! **Figure 9** shows how much more at risk you are as your T-score decreases. But remember, your T-score is only one indicator of fracture risk; other factors—like thinness, age, prior fracture, diet, exercise, and more—also contribute to your risk for breaking a bone.

The initial development of this method was based on data from White postmenopausal women, making interpretation of results less appropriate for men, premenopausal women, or non-White postmenopausal women. However, data have been collected from men and persons of varied racial/ethnic groups over time. T-scores are now calculated against a mean score developed from young normal people of the same sex as the person being tested. This method is the standard used for all postmenopausal women and men over the age of 50.

The International Society for Clinical Densitometry (ISCD) recommends using sex-matched and race- or ethnic-adjusted Z-scores for interpreting BMD test results of premenopausal women, men, and children (see Questions 32–33).

During conventional DXA testing, hip and spine measurements are taken. Depending on the brand of DXA machine, the neck of the femur (upper leg bone) or the point between the neck of the femur and the long part of the upper leg bone (intertrochanteric region) are usually measured for the hip T-score. Sometimes both are measured and the scores are averaged. The lumbar vertebrae (lower back bones) L1 to L4 are measured for the spine T-score. The lower of the two T-scores (hip or spine) is used to classify your degree of bone loss using the WHO guidelines. So, if you have a lower T-score (more bone loss) in your hip than in your spine, your hip T-score will be used for interpreting your results and making the diagnosis. **Table 2** shows an example of the results from a DXA test.

Delia's comment:

I'm used to receiving lab results that express a number that I can understand. For example, a white blood cell (WBC) count might come back as 6000 and I know that I have 6000 white blood cells in every little drop of blood, and that's pretty normal. But when I received the results of my BMD testing of my hip and spine, I was not expecting

Table 2 DXA Results

Region	BMD (g/cm²)	Young Adult (%)	Young Adult T-score	Age Matched (%)	Age Matched Z-score
Femoral Neck	0.715	73	−2.2	90	−0.6
L2–L4 (spine)	1.605	134	3.4	154	4.7

Region	Measured Date	Age (years)	BMD (g/cm²)	Change Versus Baseline (%)	Change Versus Baseline (%/yr)
Femoral Neck	02/22/2005	82.5	0.715	−0.3	−0.1
	06/05/2002	79.8	0.718	Baseline	Baseline
L2–L4	02/22/2005	82.5	1.605	2.6*	1.2*
	06/05/2002	79.8	1.549	Baseline	Baseline

T-score is based on the U.S. female reference population aged 20–40. Z-score is matched to others on age, weight, and ethnicity.

These results show that the patient (an 82-year-old White female) has osteopenia at the femoral neck of the hip (T-score of −2.2) and normal bone density at the lower spine (T-score of 3.4). Her bone density decreased at the femoral neck by a very small amount (0.3%) since her last test, but her bone density increased at the lower spine by 2.6%. The small change in bone density at the hip is not significant (e.g., it might be caused by error of the machine rather than real change), but the change at the spine is significant, meaning that she has successfully increased her bone density in that area. This report also gives the percent of change per year from current results compared to her baseline. Again, the change per year at the hip was not significant (decrease of 0.1% per year) but was significant (meaning it was not caused by measurement error, but is a real change) at the lower spine where she has had an increase of 1.2% per year since her last test. For a BMD change to be significant, it must be greater than a 2–4% change at the person's spine or a 3–6% change at the person's hip. Her Z-scores (−0.6 at the hip and 4.7 at the spine) indicate that she is close to the same bone density of others in her age group at the hip but has a higher density than others do in her age group at her spine. The Z-score results together with the T-score results suggest that she most likely has osteoporosis related to postmenopause and aging, and not due to secondary causes such as illnesses or medications.

*Indicates significant change based on 95% confidence interval

just a negative number. I was told that my spine was okay. However, I was also told that my T-score was −1.5 and therefore I had low bone mass in my hip bone. What's even more confusing is that a normal result can

Risk Factors and Testing

still be a negative number, so if I get my bone density to improve enough to be considered normal, I still might have a T-score of –0.9! That doesn't feel like very good feedback to me!

32. What is a Z-score?

A **Z-score** matches your bone mineral density with individuals of the same age, gender, and ethnicity. The following formula is used to determine your Z-score:

$$\frac{\text{Patient's BMD} - \text{BMD age-matched normal reference}}{\text{Standard deviation of age-matched reference}}$$

Z-scores are used to identify low bone mass in men under the age of 50, premenopausal women, and children. The International Society for Clinical Densitometry recommends classifying Z-scores of –2.0 and lower as "low bone mineral density for chronological age" or "below the expected range for age." They suggest classifying scores above –2.0 as "within the expected range for age." Z-scores are not helpful in identifying osteoporosis or osteopenia because your Z-score may remain constant throughout your life. Z-scores are more useful in evaluating bone density in children, who have not yet reached peak bone mass, and younger adults.

Very low Z-scores in postmenopausal women or men over 50, indicating a much lower bone mass than that of their peers, do require further investigation into the causes of bone loss related to secondary osteoporosis (the type of osteoporosis not associated with postmenopause or aging). If you have a Z-score lower than –1.5, your clinician should be looking for reasons why you have significant bone loss compared

Z-score

Matches your bone mineral density with individuals of the same age, gender, and ethnicity, and is more helpful in evaluating children and premenopausal women.

to your own age group. If you have a medical condition, for example, hyperthyroidism (one of the illnesses that can cause secondary osteoporosis) that has gone undetected, a low Z-score may point your clinician toward identifying and treating this reason for bone loss.

33. How will my clinician use my test results to determine whether I have osteoporosis?

A T-score, expressed in standard deviations, will be reported to your clinician, and your score will be evaluated using the WHO guidelines. If you are a post-menopausal woman or a man over 50, most machines are calibrated with special software to determine your scores. Based on the guidelines (see Question 31), your results will indicate normal bone density, low bone mass (osteopenia), or osteoporosis. If you have osteoporosis with a fragility fracture, you will have a diagnosis of **severe osteoporosis**. Because the T-score not only reflects bone density but also your risk of fracturing a bone, your clinician should discuss specific ways of not only increasing your bone mass but also lowering your fracture risk (see Question 79).

Severe osteoporosis
A T-score lower than −2.5 plus the presence of one or more fragility fractures.

A Z-score is usually not helpful in making the diagnosis of osteoporosis. However, if it is particularly low (lower than −1.5), it is important for your clinician to evaluate you for conditions and illnesses that may be causing your bone loss associated with secondary osteoporosis. Such causes of secondary osteoporosis might include thyroid or parathyroid disease, cigarette smoking, excessive alcohol intake, problems with absorption from your gastrointestinal tract, or the use of medications known to be harmful to bone.

If you had a peripheral bone density test (at the wrist or heel), you may still require **central testing** (at the hip or spine) even if your test results are interpreted to be in the normal range, unless you weigh over 250 pounds and a central test cannot accommodate you. Central BMD testing more accurately reflects the status of large central bones. Questions 19 and 20 identify who should have BMD screening or testing at the hip and spine, and this applies even if the test at your wrist, heel, or ankle was normal.

It's important to remember that even if your T-score fits into the category of normal, you may still have osteoporosis at another site. Even though central bones measured on a DXA are the most predictive for the rest of your body, other sites can still have lower mass. Peripheral measurements (heel, wrist) are not as predictive for the rest of your body. So, even if you have normal measures of your heel or wrist, your clinician may send you for additional testing with different machines or on other bones, especially if you have many risk factors or a fracture. If you have a frailty fracture or a low-trauma fracture (see Question 74), you likely have osteoporosis whether you are tested for it or not, although it's important to get a baseline measurement so that the effectiveness of treatment can be evaluated by your clinician.

If your T-score indicates osteoporosis according to the WHO classifications (see Question 31), the American Association of Clinical Endocrinologists (AACE) and the National Osteoporosis Foundation (NOF) recommend that your clinician complete a physical exam and laboratory analyses, such as a complete blood count (CBC) and other blood tests for minerals such as calcium and phosphorus and for liver function, kidney

Central testing

Usually DXA or QCT bone density tests of the hip, upper thigh, or spine.

It's important to remember that even if your T-score fits into the category of normal, you may still have osteoporosis at another site.

function, and electrolytes such as salt and potassium. Most clinicians also will test for your vitamin D level in the blood (serum 25-OH-D levels), fasting serum calcium level, and urinary calcium level over a 24-hour period. These additional tests will help rule out other causes for your low bone density. If other causes are identified, they can be treated so the effects on your bones are minimized (see Questions 15–16, and 47–51).

While you may be told that you have osteopenia based on your T-score, a T-score between −1.0 and −2.5 does not necessarily mean that bone loss has occurred. It could mean that you never reached peak bone mass in young adulthood to begin with. If you have osteopenia, your clinician likely will evaluate you for causes of secondary osteoporosis (see Questions 9, 15, and 16). Treatment may be indicated to prevent osteoporosis, whether the osteopenia is due to some bone loss or a low peak bone mass (Part 3 discusses treatment options). The WHO developed an algorithm to assist clinicians in determining who would benefit from initiating treatment for osteopenia, and the results from this algorithm will be included on most bone mineral density test reports by the end of 2009 (see Question 55).

34. How soon are test results usually available? Should I get a copy of the results of the testing?

Your clinician may get your bone density test results immediately, but more often than not, test results are available from 1 to 3 weeks after a test is done. You and your clinician should make a plan to discuss the results once they are available. Talking about how and when you will be informed of the results will eliminate confusion. For example, if you have normal bone

Talking about how and when you will be informed of the results will eliminate confusion.

density, will your clinician contact you? Or should you call for results? Some clinicians do not call if results are normal, so you need to be certain that your clinician has the right contact information and that "no news is good news." If your testing shows low bone mass or osteoporosis, will you need to have a follow-up visit with your clinician? Or can you discuss treatment options over the phone with your clinician?

To eliminate confusion and potential misunderstanding, when your tests are ordered, you should first determine if the clinician's office makes the testing appointment or if you must do that yourself. You should also ask your clinician when the results will be available after your scheduled test, how you will be contacted, whether a follow-up visit is required, and if so, with whom.

Some people like to have copies of their test results so that they can track their own progress, but it's not necessary to get a copy of the results of your testing. It's more important for you to know if you have osteopenia or osteoporosis so that if you must seek medical care from other providers or if you have a fall and are taken to a hospital emergency department, you will be able to inform the new providers of your diagnosis and if you are being treated.

35. If my BMD test results are normal, when should I be screened again? If my test results show either osteopenia or osteoporosis, when should my test be repeated?

If your BMD results are normal, you should be screened again 2 years after the first screening, unless your risk factors change. For example, if you develop an illness requiring that you take a steroid medication, your clinician may want to reconsider the time of your next screening. Medicare currently covers bone mineral density testing every 2 years.

Because BMD tests can be quite expensive, you may not be able to afford them if you do not have insurance to cover them. Some insurance companies will pay for retesting and monitoring based on the clinician's orders. You might be retested every 6 months to 1 year depending on your level of bone loss, your other illnesses or medications, and your treatment. If your BMD test results remain the same for two or more tests, the interval between retesting could be lengthened. You should contact the member services department of your health insurance company or HMO to get information about coverage for BMD tests. Ask when you can be screened and when you can be retested according to their guidelines. Some clinicians don't think it's necessary to monitor BMD every year because there is not enough time to show a significant difference in bone density. Most clinicians will monitor density every 2 to 3 years for those on treatment or to demonstrate stability over time. After two or more BMD tests show that bone density is not changing, a longer interval between tests is appropriate.

When you are retested to monitor the progress of treatment, keep in mind that it is important to use the same machine and preferably the same person operating the machine (who can be a nurse or technician). Each machine is calibrated differently, and keeping the same one gives more consistent results and measurable changes (see Question 69).

36. If my tests show osteoporosis in my hip, what is the likelihood that I have bone loss in other bones? Does osteoporosis ever affect the skull bone?

If your hip shows osteoporosis, it is likely that other bones have diminished bone density as well. If you are a White woman, your body singles out your hip—it loses one-third of its bone mineral density between the ages of about 30 and 80. However, other bones usually don't start to lose density until the age of menopause, or in men at a comparable age, unless you have other medical or lifestyle reasons for having osteoporosis. Approximately 4% of postmenopausal White women aged 50 to 59 have osteoporosis of the hip, and 6% of the same group have osteoporosis in the wrist. And after age 80 in postmenopausal women, osteoporosis of the hip jumps up to 52% and in the wrist to 78%! So if you are a postmenopausal woman with osteoporosis of the hip, it is very likely that you have osteoporosis of other bones, particularly the wrist.

Although you are definitely at risk for a vertebral fracture if you have been diagnosed with osteoporosis of the hip, osteoporosis of the spine is more difficult to measure because certain conditions interfere with getting accurate measurements. Measuring your spine for osteoporosis will be more difficult if you have arthritis or fractures of the spine because they interfere with the accuracy of the imaging of the spine.

More important, you will be more at risk for fracturing any bone in your body.

More important than having osteoporosis, you will be more at risk for fracturing any bone in your body. And this includes, although rarely, your skull bone. If you have been diagnosed with osteoporosis, it is critical that you take all necessary precautions to prevent falls (see Question 79).

37. What do my results say about my future risk for fracturing a bone?

Because fractures are the biggest problem associated with osteoporosis, it is important to know what your results say about your risk for fracture. It's also important to know that there is risk to fracturing your bones whether you are diagnosed with osteoporosis or not (meaning you may have it but don't know it). The lifetime risk of fracturing your hip, spine, or forearm is 40% in White women and 13% in White men. If you include the potential for fracturing other bones, your risk is increased even further. For women, the lifetime risk of fracturing a hip is equivalent to or more than the combined lifetime risk of developing breast, uterine, or ovarian cancer.

If your BMD testing shows that your bones are "normal," you are not at increased risk of fracturing a bone unless your score is between 0 and −1.0. Because scores are expressed in standard deviations, any score less than 0 represents an increased risk; the risk is small if your score is between 0 and −1.0, but it still exists.

If your T-score indicates that you have osteopenia, you could be 4 times more likely to fracture a bone. But low bone mass as defined by your T-score is not the only factor that puts you at increased risk for a fracture. Your clinician should help you understand that your age, family history of osteoporosis, previous fractures, risk of falling, and the risk of injury are other important factors when considering your risk for fracture.

As you age, your risk of fracturing any bone increases. If you are diagnosed with osteoporosis, your risk goes up even further. So if your T-score indicates that you have osteoporosis, you could be 8 times more likely

As you age, your risk of fracturing any bone increases.

to fracture a bone. If you are over 50 years of age, you have a 50% chance of suffering a fracture related to osteoporosis. And 750,000 spinal fractures occur each year. These fractures occur in people previously diagnosed with osteoporosis as well as in those who never knew they had it.

38. If my tests show I have bone loss, do I need to be referred to a specialist? Or can my primary care provider or my gynecology clinician manage my case?

Sometimes, BMD testing sites have their own clinicians. They are familiar with the BMD testing equipment and interpreting the results. You may be prescribed medication and told to follow up with them in several months. When your primary care provider (PCP) or **gynecology clinician (GYN)** orders your tests, you should discuss who will be interpreting the test results and if you will be referred to a specialist.

Most primary care providers can manage your care if you are newly diagnosed with osteoporosis or have just found out you have osteopenia. It may become necessary, depending on other medical conditions that you have or the medications you take, to refer you to a specialist in osteoporosis. This specialist is often an **endocrinologist** or **rheumatologist**.

Many women see their GYN clinician annually in place of regular primary care check-ups. GYN clinicians can order BMD testing, provide you with the results, recommend therapies and lifestyle changes, and prescribe medications. If you have other conditions that may affect your bone health, it is advisable to also have a

Gynecology clinician (GYN)

A nurse practitioner, midwife, physician assistant, or physician who specializes in the practice of gynecology, the health care of women.

Endocrinologist

Physician who specializes in the care of people with hormone disorders such as diabetes, thyroid problems, and osteoporosis.

Rheumatologist

Physician who specializes in the care of people with disorders related to joints, bones, tendons, and muscles. Unlike a surgeon, does not perform surgery on joints and bones.

primary care clinician who can review all of your medications and history as they relate to osteoporosis.

If you have spinal fractures, you may be referred to an **orthopedist** (a doctor who specializes in the treatment of the skeleton system and its muscles, joints, and **ligaments**). Although rarely used today, a special brace for your back may be recommended (see Question 83). Orthopedists usually don't prescribe the medications that are used to treat or prevent osteoporosis, unless the medication is needed for a fracture (see Question 63). Your PCP or GYN clinician usually prescribes medications for prevention and treatment. If you see different clinicians for your primary care, bone health, and GYN care, you must inform all of them about the therapies being used to manage your osteopenia or osteoporosis.

Orthopedist

A physician who specializes in the treatment and surgery of bone and joint disorders.

Ligaments

Tough bands that connect bones to each other.

39. Are there blood and urine tests that can be used to determine if I have bone loss?

In the case of osteoporosis, biochemical "markers" are chemical substances that indicate bone turnover. When osteoclasts (the cells of bone resorption; see Question 4) break down the collagen in bone, byproducts of this breakdown (for example, N-teleopeptide crosslinks [NTx]) are released into the bloodstream and excreted in the urine. When new bone is formed, byproducts such as osteocalcin and other substances also find their way to the bloodstream and get excreted in the urine. By measuring the byproducts of bone breakdown (usually in the urine) and bone formation (usually in the blood), the rate of bone turnover can be determined. If bone turnover is very rapid, like it is in women following

If bone turnover is very rapid, like it is in women following menopause, the quality of bone may be poor, thus increasing the risk of fracture.

menopause, the quality of bone may be poor, thus increasing the risk for fracture.

Currently, blood and urinary biomarkers are not used to diagnose osteoporosis, but they can be helpful in assessing how fast bone is formed and broken down. BMD testing, while important for assigning fracture risk and measuring bone mass, does not provide information about bone turnover or bone quality. Tests for biomarkers do not give any information about bone mass; however, there is some evidence that the presence of bone breakdown biomarkers in urine is associated with an increased risk of hip fracture.

While the tests are relatively simple, there is not enough consistency between tests for them to be used widely, even for monitoring the course of treatment. Research has yet to confirm that biomarkers could be used routinely to monitor the effectiveness of treatment. There is some evidence based on urinary biomarkers, however, that individuals with high bone turnover have the best response to certain treatments, and those with reduced amounts of the markers, which indicate bone resorption (breakdown), also had fewer vertebral fractures. Other research demonstrates that urine biomarkers can show bone's response to medications in as little as 6 weeks, which is much faster than the traditional follow-up BMD testing done after 1 to 2 years of treatment. The future hope is that medications for osteoporosis could be changed to different ones more quickly if bone weren't responding in the intended way, based on the urinary biomarkers.

PART THREE

Lifestyle Changes and Treatments

After I'm diagnosed with osteoporosis or told that I have osteopenia, what happens next?

I understand that exercise is important for the treatment of osteoporosis. Why?

My clinician has encouraged me to take calcium supplements. There are so many kinds of calcium. How do I know I'm taking the right kind and the right amount?

More...

40. After I'm diagnosed with osteoporosis or told that I have osteopenia, what happens next?

Once you have been sent for BMD testing, it's a good idea to investigate management options for osteopenia and osteoporosis. If your results are abnormal, you and your clinician can select the regimen that you both feel is best suited for your individual case. If your testing results come back in the normal range, you will still need to discuss prevention of osteoporosis to keep your bones healthy. If your T-score shows that you have osteopenia or osteoporosis, secondary causes of osteoporosis should be ruled out before treatments are suggested.

It is very difficult to fully reverse osteoporosis once it is present.

You might think that after you are told you have osteopenia or are diagnosed with osteoporosis, your only goal should be to get rid of it. That is not the case. It is very difficult to fully reverse osteoporosis once it is present, but there are several important goals that you will want to work with your clinician to achieve:

• Reduce the risk of fracture. Although the bones in your spine can fracture without warning or trauma, fractures are most often associated with falls. It is important to change your environment and lifestyle to prevent falls so that the risk of fracture is minimized (see Question 79). You will also need to adjust your exercise routine to avoid bending your spine too far forward (see Question 44).

• Relieve symptoms of fractures and/or skeletal deformity. This may require pain medications and a change in your exercise routine. Question 84 discusses exercises that may help minimize the deformity from kyphosis.

- Improve mobility, activity level, and ability to function despite fractures or the potential for fractures. An in-home assessment by staff from a home health agency may be helpful in evaluating your risk for fractures. They can also explain how you can change your environment so that you can maintain or improve your mobility and avoid falls. If you have fractured a bone, you will need to maintain your body strength by continuing to exercise. If you have fractured your spine (vertebral bones) or your hip, the tendency may be to isolate yourself from others and become home bound. It is an important goal of treatment to maintain social connections, despite bone loss or the presence of fractures.
- Prevent further bone loss. You don't want to lose any more bone than you already have. Make lifestyle changes that will aid in reducing further bone loss.
- Maintain the integrity of bone. You will want to be especially thoughtful about having a healthy diet. Consider carefully the amount of calcium, vitamin D, and other nutrients you are taking in to make strong bones. You will also need to do appropriate exercises.
- Regulate bone turnover. The goal is for bone formation to stay equal to or ahead of bone breakdown. Although this goal might be accomplished with lifestyle changes, regulating bone turnover may require prescription medication.

It is important to remember that your goals toward improving or maintaining good bone health will require lifelong effort. You won't feel medications working. You won't know if your bones are responding until you have follow-up testing. So, after you've been told you have osteopenia or have been diagnosed with osteoporosis, remember to:

- Maintain a positive attitude about your diagnosis.
- Read as much as you can about osteopenia and osteoporosis.
- Develop a management regimen with your clinician—one that you can live with.
- Use the suggestions in this book and the resources in Appendix B to develop a healthy lifestyle.
- Think of this as a beginning—not an end—to good bones and an active life. It is never too late to improve your bone health!

41. What if I am told that I have osteopenia but not osteoporosis?

If you have osteopenia, then your T-score is 1 to 2.5 standard deviations below the bone density of the average healthy young adult. Given a score in that range, your bone mass is somewhere between 10% and 30% below normal for a young adult, and your risk of fracture, based on your T-score alone, is as much as 2 to 5 times that of a healthy young adult with normal bone density. Therefore, it's still important to prevent falls.

Sometimes clinicians don't use the term osteopenia. Instead, they prefer to tell patients they have low bone mass.

Although your T-score may indicate that you have osteopenia, it is best to assume that your bone loss will continue if you do not embrace the goals and behaviors intended to improve your bone health. Sometimes clinicians don't use the term osteopenia. Instead, they prefer to tell patients that they have low bone mass. Some clinicians may suggest prescription medications specifically intended to prevent further bone loss or to increase bone density. However, management options for osteopenia have been controversial, and some clinicians think prescription medications for osteopenia are not appropriate. See Question 55 for more about medications for osteoporosis and who should be treated. In either case and whether you have lost bone mass or not, your clinician should always emphasize the importance of calcium, vitamin D, and appropriate exercise.

Finding out that you have osteopenia represents an opportunity. While no one wants to have low bone mass, you have an opportunity to avoid developing osteoporosis. Even if your clinician doesn't prescribe medications for you, you can still make behavioral changes that can make the difference between having osteopenia and going on to develop osteoporosis.

So, now that you have been told you have osteopenia, what can you do to change your lifestyle to make it more bone-friendly? There are several things that you can do now, no matter what your age:

- Calculate your intake of calcium and vitamin D, making sure that you are getting the necessary amount every day (see Questions 47 and 51).
- Get moving. Exercise can help slow the rate of bone loss by increasing the rate of bone formation. Consistent, moderate exercise is associated with a big decrease in hip fractures. Remember that bone strength increases in your body at the location where you exercise. For example, walking benefits the lower spine, hips, and leg bones but not the arms or upper back (see Question 42).
- Stop smoking.
- If, on average, you drink more than one or two alcoholic drinks per day (one serving of alcohol is 5 ounces of wine, 12 ounces of beer, or one cocktail containing 1.5 ounces of hard liquor), cut back or avoid alcohol entirely.

While no one wants to have low bone mass, you have an opportunity to avoid developing osteoporosis.

Lifestyle Changes and Treatments

- Drink water, milk, or calcium-enriched beverages instead of coffee and soda. If you drink coffee, add milk to add some calcium. Large amounts of caffeine can interfere with calcium absorption. However, if you are getting an adequate amount of calcium, moderate caffeine intake (1–2 cups/day) is unlikely to cause a problem. Large amounts of phosphorus can also interfere with calcium, but you would have to consume more than 3 to 4 grams of phosphorus per day for phosphorus to be a problem.

Question 86 discusses dietary changes to lessen or avert the effects of osteoporosis and osteopenia.

42. I understand that exercise is important for the treatment of osteoporosis. Why?

It doesn't matter how old you are—exercise is important to your overall health. An increase in exercise can decrease your risk of heart disease, high blood pressure, diabetes, breast cancer, and colon cancer. Exercise will give you more energy and better sleep. Regular exercise has also been found to decrease depression in a couple of ways. First, exercise releases endorphins, the "feel-good" substances related to mood. Second, the social interaction of group exercise or sports can reduce depression as well.

We can add bone health to the list of important reasons to exercise because we know that the stress of weight-bearing exercise and strength training helps bone mass. Any significant increases in stress on bone from exercise—that is, weight-bearing and resistance exercises—will actually signal the need to build more bone. Stress on bone literally shifts the bone-building process into high gear. Exercise is known to assist individuals who want to lose weight or who want to maintain a healthy weight, and exercise may also play a role in reducing symptoms of arthritis (see Question 96). Strength training exercises, such as weight lifting, can increase your body's muscle mass, which in turn increases your body's metabolic rate. If you increase your muscle mass by 3 pounds, your metabolic rate increases by 7%, which allows you to add some extra calories to your diet without fearing they will add extra fat.

Exercise is important in preventing and treating osteoporosis for several reasons. First, it improves the integrity of the bone by preserving what you already have. The stress on bone that is exerted by weight-bearing and resistance exercise causes an increase in bone formation. Secondly, exercise can help to reduce falls by improving muscle tone and balance. Lastly, though definitely not least in the order of importance, moderate weight-bearing exercise for 4 hours per week can reduce the risk of hip fracture by up to 40%.

The less you engage in physical activity, the less stress is placed on your bones. This costs you bone mass and muscle mass, a high price to pay for a sedentary lifestyle. Women engage in regular physical activity less than men, and they can ill afford to be less active because they are at higher risk of osteoporosis just by virtue of being women. Inadequate activity can make anyone, but particularly women, become frail, increasing their risk of osteoporosis and fracture.

Marjory's comment:

As a nurse, I've always been aware of when my rheumatologist was examining my hands and feet for bone density

Inadequate activity can make anyone, but particularly women, become frail, increasing their risk of osteoporosis and fracture.

and evidence of rheumatoid arthritis, he said my bones looked good and that I didn't have osteoporosis. I had my first bone density test of my hip and spine about 10 years ago, and I've had a couple more since then. After one of the tests, my doctor said that I had the bones of a 27-year-old (but where did the body of the 27-year-old go?!). I try to maintain a healthy diet with lots of fruits and vegetables, but I also know I should lose about 20 pounds. It's just that the one disadvantage to exercising regularly is that it makes me so hungry! In addition to exercising regularly, I take 1000 mg of calcium supplements with vitamin D. And, in part because I was getting lots of foot cramps in the pool and at night, I also take 500 mg a day of magnesium.

43. What types of exercises should I do, and how often?

If you have been leading a sedentary lifestyle, start an exercise program after you have discussed it with your clinician. Then, start by changing your attitude first. Do small things that will change your activity level. Park your car further away from your destination than you usually do. Take stairs instead of elevators (do this gradually—stairs can be very tough if you're out of shape). Walk more briskly than usual while shopping. Take a short walk after lunch instead of eating an extra cookie (see Question 45).

Aerobic exercise

Type of activity intended to strengthen the heart, such as running, cycling, or brisk walking, by increasing your breathing and heart rate; helps the body to burn off fat and control cholesterol.

There are two types of exercise that can help to improve your bone health: weight-bearing and resistive.

There are two types of exercise that can help to improve your bone health: weight-bearing and resistive. Weight-bearing exercises are those that literally require supporting or carrying weight and include walking, running, **aerobics**, hiking, stair climbing, dancing, tennis, jumping rope, and kick-boxing, among others. Basketball, soccer, jumping rope, and hiking, while good exercise, can cause more falls due to the likelihood of contact with other players or slipping. Kick-boxing can pose risks for fractures with contact as well. Due to these risks, kick-boxing, basketball, soccer, jumping rope, and hiking may not be the best choices for people with osteoporosis. If you have access to snow, cross-country skiing and snow-shoeing are also excellent weight-bearing activities. Resistive exercises mean that you are pushing or pulling against weight or force; thus the activity causes resistance to your muscles and bones. Resistive exercises include activities like swimming, biking, cycling, stationary biking, **Pilates, tai chi**, **yoga**, rowing, canoeing, and weight-training. Regular swimming and street biking by themselves are not effective for strengthening bone. However, continually increasing resistance while swimming or biking and coupling these activities with other exercises that increase stress or load will strengthen bone.

In order for exercise to be effective, you must provide more "load" than your bones are accustomed to carrying. So, for weight-bearing exercise, you must continually increase the duration or the amount of impact of the exercises. For resistive exercises, you should continually, but gradually, add resistance: increase the weights that you lift; increase the resistance on your stationary bike; or swim longer, use water barbells, or do more vigorous water exercises. Once you stop exercising, the benefits to your bones stop as well. You will begin to lose bone mass with a measurable decrease in bone density in as little as 1 month. Remember, all physical activity is still good, though, whether its effects build bone, strengthen muscles, improve flexibility and balance, enhance mood and self-esteem, or help you to sleep better.

Pilates

A type of activity for muscles that promotes strength and flexibility; developed by Joseph Pilates, this group of exercises can be done by yourself or in a class.

Tai chi

A form of exercise that combines meditation and flexibility training.

Yoga

A group of breathing exercises and movements intended to improve flexibility and strength, and bring about tranquility.

There is ongoing debate in the scientific community about how much and how often exercise must be done in order to be effective. There is general agreement that 30 minutes of exercise three times per week is the minimum required to maintain bone integrity. However, the latest dietary guidelines from the United States Department of Agriculture (USDA) and the United States Department of Health and Human Services (DHHS) advise 60 minutes of moderately vigorous exercise daily or most days in order to maintain good overall health. But don't overdo it! Running for more than 5 hours per week has been related to lower bone mass, and any exercising that leads to amenorrhea (absence of menstrual periods) should also be avoided.

If you are unable to tolerate weight-lifting or do not have access to weights at a gym, there are chair exercises that you can do. Appendix A shows some of the exercises that you can do without having to go to a gym. If you have access to a stationary bike, you can use this as resistive exercise, at least for your legs. Some stationary bikes have handles that allow you to push your arms back and forth while cycling, providing resistance to your arms and upper body. It is important to increase the resistance setting over time to increase the load on your muscles and bones.

Before you engage in a new exercise program, it's important that you consult your clinician, particularly if you have recently been diagnosed with any new illness or condition, or have been placed on new medication. Even though you may be enthusiastic about changing your activity level, it's important to change your level gradually. If you have never been on a treadmill, don't start your new routine by trying to run miles at a time. You should not jump into a weight-training program by lifting excessive weight or doing too many repetitions. You will end up sore and discouraged. Start out slowly but maintain a consistent schedule. Commit to exercising at least 3 days per week. You should not weight-lift 2 days in a row. Your muscles need time to rest between sessions.

Remember that exercise without getting enough calcium and vitamin D will not help your bones (see Questions 47–51). Similarly, exercise must incorporate both weight-bearing and resistance to help strengthen bone. Exercise works best to increase bone density for women when you are premenopausal or if you are taking estrogen. But that is not to say that you shouldn't exercise if you are postmenopausal and not taking hormones. In fact, the results of the Nurses' Health Study showed that walking 8 hours per week was comparable to taking hormones to protect against fractures in postmenopausal women.

If you have kyphosis (see Question 85), there are some exercises that you can do to reduce the amount of curve you have as well as strengthen the muscles around your spine. The goal is to do exercises that extend your spine and strengthen your abdominal, erector, spinal, and scapular muscles. Question 85 discusses which exercises can help you, and Appendix A contains appropriate exercises for strengthening your muscles.

Marjory's comment:

Water aerobics is a wonderful form of exercise. Even before my knee replacements, water took away almost all of the pain. Although I needed to take anti-inflammatory medications for pain, I was really quite comfortable in the water. Now I go to my water aerobics class 4 times per week. We do cross-country ski movements, jumping jacks, rolls, and knees-to-nose exercises, all in deep water wearing a flotation belt. There is no jarring on my joints, and a warm water pool feels great. I am not able to do any kneeling when it comes to exercise, so exercise in the water fits with what I'm able to do. We do exercises to help our back muscles get strong so that we can have straighter backs, too. Water aerobics is also a social activity because the instructor makes sure we all know each other by first names before she gets started with the class, where we only see one another from the neck up. Then when we see each other in the grocery store we raise a few eyebrows from onlookers by saying, "Oh, I didn't recognize you with your clothes on!"

44. Are there any exercises that I should avoid? Yoga and tai chi are great exercises, but are they helpful for preventing or treating osteoporosis?

If you have never skied, ice skated, or roller bladed, don't start now! In fact, any sport or exercise that involves the possibility of falling is not a good one for those trying to preserve their bones. Contact sports can be a problem. Golf and bowling can cause too much bending and twisting of the spine and could be more harmful than helpful.

If you have been diagnosed with either osteoporosis or a vertebral fracture, forward bending (**flexion**) is also a bad idea whether you are exercising or not. **Figure 10** shows the body positions and exercises that you should avoid. You will probably recognize that these positions are related to exercises such as toe-touches and sit-ups. When you bend forward, you are pressing the front, or anterior, parts of the vertebrae, causing them to "crunch," or compress. This kind of compression can cause fractures. Figure 6 (Question 18) shows how tiny

Flexion

A bending motion of any joint.

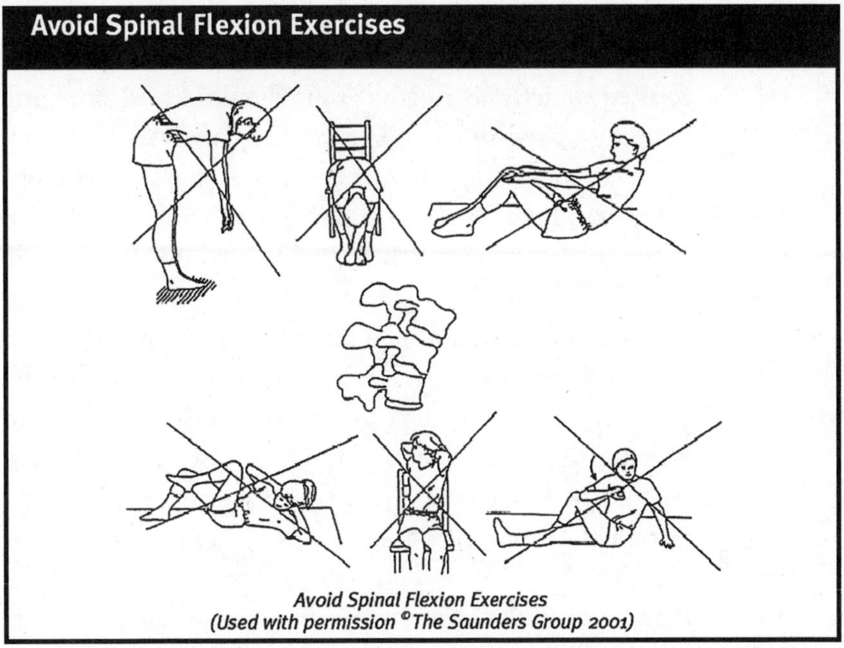

Avoid Spinal Flexion Exercises

Avoid Spinal Flexion Exercises
(Used with permission ©The Saunders Group 2001)

Figure 10   Positions and movements to avoid when exercising if you have osteoporosis.
Source: Duke University Medical Center's Bone and Metabolic Disease Clinic. Reprinted with permission. Gold DT, Lee LS, Tresolini CP, eds. *Working with Patients to Prevent, Treat, and Manage Osteoporosis: A Curriculum Guide for the Health Professions*, **3rd ed. Durham, NC: Center for the Study of Aging and Human Development, Duke University Medical Center; 2001.**

fractures eventually cause the spine to bend forward in a curve (kyphosis). In one study of women with osteoporosis, 89% of women who regularly did spinal flexion exercises also developed at least one new vertebral fracture.

You should also avoid rotation of the spine. For example, do not do alternating toe-touches where you touch your hand to the opposite foot. Some weight-lifting machines provide for exercising the muscles near the waist by holding the lower body steady and twisting the upper body with weights. Avoid this type of rotation exercise if you have osteoporosis of the spine.

Some of the positions of yoga and tai chi are not appropriate for people with osteoporosis unless they are performed exactly correctly. You should avoid forward bending or twisting of the spine. In yoga, the goal is to bend at the waist while keeping the back completely straight, but since most people do not bend at the waist without also bending their spine, forward bending in yoga is not advised. Yoga and tai chi are both excellent exercises for flexibility and stretching, and for gradually straightening limbs and spine to their full **extension**, however. They are also great for stress management because they both use a combination of breathing and smooth body movements. If you regularly practice yoga or tai chi, you are also more likely to have good balance and therefore prevent falls. And a recent study indicated that yoga might also help to prevent weight gain at midlife. This added benefit is most likely because those who regularly practice yoga seem to be more in tune with their bodies and experience less stress, depression, or boredom that can lead to poor eating habits.

Learning good body mechanics without bending or twisting the spine is important. Activities of daily living such as making your bed, putting clothes or food away on lower shelves, and even removing food from the oven can cause vertebral fractures if you have osteoporosis. Bending at the knees without forward flexion of your spine will keep the pressure off the front edges of your spine bones. It's also important to distribute your weight evenly over your knees when you bend them to avoid twisting or rotation of the spine. Bending forward with heavy groceries or anything heavy can be particularly dangerous to your spine.

Exercise is site-specific. This means that if you exercise your forearms and wrists, the bone density in your

Extension

Straightening a flexed limb.

If you regularly practice yoga or tai chi, you are also more likely to have good balance and therefore prevent falls.

wrist and forearm will improve, but not in other bones. Your bones only get stronger in the areas where you are exercising. And if you stop exercising routinely, the improvement in your bones will be lost.

45. I'm 60 years old and was recently diagnosed with osteoporosis. I've never exercised regularly, but I've heard that walking is the best exercise for someone like me. Is that true?

Because you are still able to walk and have not exercised regularly, walking is the best form of exercise for you to start with. In 2001, as part of his report on obesity, the United States Surgeon General urged that all Americans adopt the habit of taking 10,000 or more steps every day. This number was based on the need to get at least 30 minutes of exercise over and above your normal daily activities. The researchers came up with 10,000 steps as a reasonable goal to get America moving. And walking is free!

So, to get started with a walking program that will benefit your bones, your heart, your weight, and your overall health, try the following:

- Consult your clinician to make sure that a new walking program is appropriate for you and that you don't have any limitations for medical reasons.
- Make sure that you are doing other things to prevent further bone loss, like cutting down on alcohol and stopping cigarette smoking. If you don't get enough calcium and vitamin D, even vigorous exercise and walking will not help your bones.

- Find a friend who will partner with you. Walking with a friend can be good for both of you. And if you make a commitment to walk together, you are more likely to accomplish your daily goal.

- Buy a **pedometer**. Make sure that you wear it clipped to your waistband or belt so that it will be an accurate reflection of your steps. Keep track of the number of steps you are currently taking. You may find that you are taking anywhere from 900 to 3000 steps per day, depending on the usual level of your activity.

- Your goal is 10,000 steps per day. If your normal activities only allow 2000 steps per day, you will need to walk an additional 8000 steps. But don't do all of that right away!

- Gradually add a few hundred steps to your total and try to walk that number every day for about 2 weeks. Then add a few hundred more steps.

- If you get chest pain, become overly tired, have shortness of breath, or feel weak or dizzy at any point, stop immediately and contact your clinician or emergency services. If you develop pain in your muscles or joints, you may be overdoing the walking. Inflammation in the muscles supporting the shin bone of your lower leg (tibia) is called "shin splints." Contrary to popular belief, shin splints are not tiny fractures of the shin bone, but they do result from excessive weight-bearing exercise and occur more frequently in those with flat feet. **Plantar fasciitis** (inflammation that causes pain on the sole of your foot) can be caused by the repetitive motion of walking and pounding your feet. Rest up and decrease the number of steps in your day until you are feeling better. Some fitness experts recommend stretching exercises before and after walking to avoid pain in your shins, knees, and hips. Stretching should be

Pedometer

A small gadget that measures the number of footsteps taken.

Plantar fasciitis

An inflammation of the connective tissue of the bottom of the foot, which can cause severe pain.

done gently and just until you feel a stretch, but never bounce. Anything more than gentle stretching causes too much stress on the body's ligaments. If you are unable to continue walking without pain or discomfort, contact your clinician.

- When you are walking for exercise on the street, around a track, or on a treadmill, it is very important to have comfortable shoes with good support. Replace sneakers about every 6 months or sooner if you notice they are wearing out.

- Drink water. Staying hydrated even if you're walking in a comfortable temperature is important.

- Maintain good posture while walking. There is often a tendency to walk with your head down. Try to keep your shoulders back and aligned over your hips, your head up, and for even more of a challenge, keep your abdominal muscles pulled in.

- Once you are well established in your walking program, you can start to add small hand weights. Begin with 1-pound weights for each hand (or a 16-ounce bottle of water in each hand). You can even add ankle weights to make your walking more challenging once you've reached a level where you are comfortable. It's important to consistently increase the load on your bones, and adding hand weights will also benefit your arms and upper back.

- There are audio CDs and tapes that can make your walking routine more fun and challenging by adding alternate exercises and music. It's important to stay interested and engaged in walking, and it's an exercise you can do almost anywhere.

- Be safe. If you walk in the evening or early morning before dawn, be sure to wear reflective tape on your clothing or sneakers. If you walk during the winter, avoid icy sidewalks so that you won't fall. If you use headphones, be alert to traffic and your surroundings.

46. I have been in postmenopause for 5 years. I've always been faithful about exercise, weight-training, and taking my calcium, and yet I've recently been told that I have osteopenia. Why didn't doing these things prevent bone loss? What more can I do?

Being postmenopausal is the most significant risk factor for having osteopenia and osteoporosis. Don't forget that if you are postmenopausal, you may lose about 2% to 5% of your bone mass per year for the first 4 to 8 years following menopause. Because you are between 4 and 8 years postmenopause, you are experiencing the time of greatest bone loss.

Even with the explanation of being postmenopausal, it can feel pretty discouraging if it seems like you're doing all the right things but you find out you have bone loss anyway. This doesn't mean that you are doing anything wrong. And you absolutely should not stop exercising and taking your calcium and vitamin D. Your healthy habits may not have prevented osteopenia for several reasons.

First, look back at your pattern of growth and food intake. Were you very thin as a child and adolescent? Did you drink enough milk and eat plenty of dairy products? Was your diet overall a healthy one with a good balance of protein, carbohydrates, and fats, without a lot of junk food, soda, and coffee? If you were excessively thin; if you did not get enough calcium, vitamin D, and other nutrients; if you smoked; or if you consumed excessive amounts of caffeine- and phosphorus-containing foods and beverages that replaced those with calcium, it is possible that you did not reach peak bone mass as a young adult. Therefore, your T-score may reflect a failure to reach peak bone mass rather than loss of bone mass as a midlife adult.

Second, what is your family history? If you have a first-degree relative (mother, father, sister, brother, daughter, son) with osteoporosis, you are much more likely to have osteopenia or osteoporosis even if you've done everything you can to prevent bone loss.

Third, do you have other risk factors besides family history that may have contributed to the condition of your bones? For example, if you are on steroids for chronic asthma or other medical conditions, significant loss of bone density can happen in as little as 3 weeks. Unfortunately, steroid use can create loss of bone density faster than exercise and calcium can increase it.

And fourth, are there lifestyle changes that you should be making? You already exercise and take calcium, but you should also quit smoking and cut down on alcohol if you are consuming more than one or two drinks per day.

Regardless of how you happened to be diagnosed with osteopenia, you will need to discuss goals and treatment with your clinician. Even though there are other reasons why you may have sustained bone loss, you should also reexamine your exercise regimen. Are you gradually and consistently increasing load on your bones?

And have another look at your calcium supplementation to make sure you are correctly calculating how much calcium you are taking in through diet and supplements. Add more calcium if you are not getting enough (see Question 47). Prescription medications may prevent further bone loss (see Question 55).

You have a chance to make some real changes in your life based on that one bone density test, so take advantage of this opportunity. There's always more we can do to get and stay healthy.

47. My clinician has encouraged me to take calcium supplements. There are so many kinds of calcium. How do I know I'm taking the right kind and the right amount?

Calcium is one of the cornerstones of developing and maintaining healthy bones. It is important to get adequate calcium in your diet, no matter how old you are. **Table 3** lists the amount of calcium recommended for your age and gender. Your daily intake should never exceed 2500 mg of elemental calcium.

Before your clinician can recommend calcium supplementation, you will need to calculate the amount of calcium you take in through your diet on a daily basis. **Table 4** shows the many different dietary sources of calcium. If you have a reasonably healthy diet, you can make it easy on yourself by using a simple formula to determine how much calcium you will need to supplement what you are getting in food. The formula goes like this: Take the number of dairy servings that you eat or drink every day and multiply that number by 300. Add 290 if you are female, or if you are male and over the age of 60; add 370 if you are a male under 60 (an expected amount of calcium from all other dietary sources except supplements). Then subtract that total from the recommended daily allowance (RDA) that is correct for your age and sex (see Table 3). The remainder is the number of milligrams of elemental calcium that you should add through supplements.

Table 3   Daily Calcium Requirements by Age and Sex

Age and Gender	Adequate Daily Intake of Calcium
Infants male or female 0–6 months	210 mg
Infants male or female 7–12 months	270 mg
Children male or female 1–3 years	500 mg
Children male or female 4–8 years	800 mg
Males and females 9–18 years	1300 mg
Males and females* 19–50 years	1000 mg
Males and females** 51 years and older	1200 mg
Pregnant or lactating female 14–18 years	1300 mg
Pregnant or lactating female 19–50 years	1000 mg

*If you are female and in menopause, you should increase your calcium intake to 1200 mg.
**Some clinicians recommend 1500 mg of calcium per day for postmenopausal women.
Source: National Academy of Sciences

Formula for all women and for men over 60:

RDA – (300 × number of daily dairy servings) + 290
= Total number of milligrams of elemental calcium
you need to take in supplements.

Formula for men under the age of 60:

RDA – (300 × number of daily dairy servings) + 370
= Total number of milligrams of elemental calcium
you need to take in supplements.

Table 4 Food Sources of Calcium

Food Source	Serving Size	Calcium Amount
Tofu (with calcium sulfate)	½ cup	434 mg
Milk, skim	1 cup	321 mg
Yogurt, low fat	1 cup	300 mg
Calcium-fortified orange juice	8 oz	300 mg
Milk, whole	1 cup	291 mg
Milk, whole, chocolate	1 cup	280 mg
Swiss cheese	1 slice	270 mg
Collard greens (cooked)	1 cup	226 mg
Monterey Jack cheese	1 slice	210 mg
Canned sardines (with bones)**	3 oz	204 mg
Cheddar cheese	1 slice	200 mg
Canned salmon (with bones)**	3 oz	181 mg
Broccoli	1 cup	180 mg
American processed cheese	1 slice	174 mg
Mozzarella cheese	1 slice	174 mg
Yogurt, frozen	½ cup	152 mg
Bread (calcium-fortified)	1 slice	150 mg
Turnip greens (cooked)	1 cup	147 mg
Cottage cheese	1 cup	140 mg

Table 4   Food Sources of Calcium (*cont.*)

Food Source	Serving Size	Calcium Amount
Mustard greens	1 cup	103 mg
Almonds	¼ cup	92 mg
Ice cream	½ cup	75 mg
Cereal (calcium-fortified)	1 cup	Varies

*Spinach and Swiss chard have binders that can interfere with calcium absorption, and most green leafy vegetables provide only a very small amount of calcium in the diet due to poor absorption.
**Calcium content includes eating the bones.

Here's the tricky part. Not all forms of calcium are created equal. The kind of calcium that your body can absorb and use is called **elemental calcium**. So the calcium in your regular diet is elemental calcium because it occurs naturally in the foods you eat and drink. The kind of calcium that is added to food is different from the type of calcium that is found naturally in foods.

When you are deciding how much calcium you need to supplement your dietary intake, you have to be aware that the different forms of calcium provide different amounts of elemental calcium (the kind that your body can absorb and use). **Table 5** shows how the different types of calcium provide different percentages of elemental calcium.

You need to look at supplement labels carefully, as many now list the elemental calcium that your body can actually absorb. For example, both Citracal® and Tums list the elemental calcium per serving, and a serving is usually two tablets. Similar to foods, elemental

Elemental calcium

The calcium that your body absorbs and uses.

Lifestyle Changes and Treatments

97

Table 5   Types of Calcium Supplements

Type of Calcium	Amount of Elemental Calcium	Amount of Elemental Calcium Absorbed per 1000 mg**	Sample Product Names
Calcium carbonate*	40.0%	400 mg	Tums, Os-Cal, Calci-Fresh Gum®, Viactiv, many others
Calcium phosphate tribasic	37.5%	375 mg	Posture, fortified products
Calcium citrate*	21.1%	211 mg	Citracal, Calci-Fresh Gum
Calcium gluconate	9.0%	90 mg	Various; often mixed with other mineral and calcium supplements
Calcium glubionate	6.4%	64 mg	Neo-Calglucon syrup

*Most frequently used supplements
**Many manufacturers now list the elemental calcium in their product per one serving, which is often two tablets. (For example, if you are taking two tablets that contain 750 mg of calcium carbonate each, you can absorb 600 mg of elemental calcium. The label will say 600 mg calcium per serving because one serving is two tablets. If you take two tablets that contain 1500 mg of calcium citrate each, you can absorb 630 mg of elemental calcium; the label will say 630 mg calcium per serving because one serving is two tablets.) The easiest way to determine if the label is listing elemental calcium is to see how it relates to the suggested daily amount. The suggested daily amount is based on 1000 mg of elemental calcium (even though many people need more than that). If the label says there is 630 mg per serving (or two tablets) and the amount listed is 63% of the suggested daily amount, you know it is elemental calcium because 630 mg is 63% of 1000 mg.

calcium amounts are based on a recommended intake of 1000 mg per day (even though intake requirements vary by age and sex). So if a serving provides 600 mg of elemental calcium, the supplement label will also note that it provides 60% of the recommended daily intake.

Because calcium supplements are manufactured in other forms besides tablets, you have more options for getting the right amount of calcium in your diet. This means that if you can't swallow big tablets, you can use chewable tablets or candy, liquid, or gum, or drink fortified orange juice.

When you buy calcium supplements, you will need to read the label so that you can get the type that is best for you:

- *Calcium carbonate* is the most commonly manufactured form of calcium. It comes in tablets that you swallow whole, chewable tablets, soft-gel tablets, liquid, flavored chewy candies, and even chewing gum. Calcium carbonate is best absorbed in an acidic environment, so it should be taken with meals. The main drawbacks to calcium carbonate are constipation and the gastrointestinal gas it can cause. To avoid excessive rumblings, discomfort, and flatulence, try taking it with a preparation that also contains magnesium. Tums, Viactiv®, Os-Cal®, and Mylanta are all examples of calcium carbonate.
- *Calcium citrate* is better tolerated and doesn't need the high level of acid from your stomach that calcium carbonate does for absorption, so it can be taken at bedtime or on an empty stomach. Calcium citrate, which comes in tablets and liquid, is a good option for people who tend to have heartburn or chronic stomach upset and for those who take medication to reduce stomach acid. Citracal is an example of calcium citrate.
- *Calcium phosphate* is most often found in fortified beverages like orange juice or by itself in a product called Posture®. Calcium phosphate does not usually cause stomach upset.
- *Calcium gluconate* and *calcium glubionate* are less commonly used because they have relatively low levels of absorbable elemental calcium. Neo-Calglucon Syrup® is an example of calcium glubionate. Calcium gluconate is sometimes combined with calcium carbonate in certain products and vitamin preparations.

It may feel like you need a math degree in order to get the right amount of calcium, but once you find the calcium that you like and can tolerate, stick with it and try to take the same number of tablets, chews, or liquid every day. Don't forget to add in what you may also take in through a daily vitamin and antacids, both of which commonly contain some form of calcium. As long as you don't go over the maximum of 2500 mg of elemental calcium per day, don't worry about getting too much.

Besides keeping your bones healthy, calcium has many other benefits:

- It builds and maintains strong teeth.
- It can lower the risk of breast cancer (if you're pre-menopausal).
- It may reduce the risk of prostate cancer.
- It can reduce the risk of colon cancer.
- When combined with magnesium, it can reduce the occurrence of headaches.
- It can reduce premenstrual syndrome (PMS) symptoms.
- It may reduce the number of hot flashes experienced by peri- and postmenopausal women.
- It can help you lose weight!
- It maintains the mineral balance in all other organs, including your brain and heart, keeping your mental function healthy and your blood pressure normal.
- It helps with muscle contractions and relaxation.
- It helps your blood clot appropriately.
- It helps to regulate hormone secretion.

Keeping up with your calcium is a win-win situation, for both your bones and your overall health.

Keeping up with your calcium is a win-win situation, for both your bones and your overall health.

Recently, coral calcium has been touted as a cure-all for many diseases as well as the best source of calcium.

Coral calcium is believed to be taken from the Japanese island of Okinawa where people are thought to live much longer than the rest of the world's peoples. Calcium manufactured from sea coral or hard shell sea creatures, however, is actually calcium carbonate, the same calcium that is available and less costly in many calcium supplements. Don't be misled by the claims that coral calcium can cure you of many diseases, even cancer and **Alzheimer's disease**.

48. What foods can I eat to assure that I'm getting enough calcium?

A diet rich in calcium will make it less likely that you will need calcium supplementation. Dairy sources of calcium include milk (all types, from skim to whole to buttermilk), yogurt, and cheese (varies with type). It is important to check the serving size of the food you're eating. For example, Table 4 (Question 47) lists foods in descending order by the amount of calcium they contain. You will note that 8 ounces of low-fat plain yogurt contain 300 mg of calcium, but when you go to the supermarket, yogurt may be sold in a 6-ounce container, giving you less calcium.

Instead of listing the amount of calcium (in mg), sometimes nutrition labels list the percentage of calcium that the food provides toward your recommended daily allowance (RDA). This RDA is actually based on 1000 mg of calcium. So if a nutrition label says you are getting 30% of your daily amount of calcium, you are getting 300 mg. But if you are postmenopausal, that is only about 20% of the RDA for you.

Cheese presents an interesting comparison of calcium amounts. You have to eat 1 cup of cottage cheese to get

Alzheimer's disease
Degenerative brain disorder that gradually causes disorientation, confusion, and memory loss.

A diet rich in calcium will make it less likely that you will need calcium supplementation.

Lifestyle Changes and Treatments

the same amount of calcium in $\frac{1}{4}$ cup of part-skim mozzarella. As much as we would all love to credit ice cream with being a great source of calcium, there is generally only about 85 mg of calcium in a $\frac{1}{2}$ cup serving. That's not a good source, because it provides only about 6% of your required amount of elemental calcium but adds up to 170 calories to your daily calorie intake.

If you are lactose intolerant, you may need to be especially careful about getting adequate calcium because most calcium in a normal diet comes from dairy sources. But you can still get adequate amounts of calcium from such foods as tofu (soybean curd), salmon, and sardines (with bones). Eating calcium-fortified cereal and orange juice will help increase your calcium intake without consuming dairy products.

49. When should I take calcium supplements? Is there any particular time of day that makes calcium more effective? Should I take it before meals, with meals, or between meals?

Depending on the type of calcium supplements you take, you may want to adjust the time of taking them. Because calcium carbonate tends to cause more stomach upset and needs stomach acid to be absorbed, it's best to take it immediately after a meal. Calcium citrate can be taken any time.

Although calcium carbonate is generally absorbed best after meals, there are some substances and foods that can interfere with the absorption of any type of calcium.

For example, too much fiber in your diet can slow the rate at which calcium is absorbed by your body. However, a high-fiber diet has also been associated with healthful changes, such as decreased risks of breast and colon cancer. Increasing fiber in your diet can also decrease the constipation associated with calcium carbonate. Dividing the amount of calcium that you need into smaller doses to take throughout the day may provide better absorption and fewer side effects of bloating and gas.

High levels of protein can also interfere with calcium absorption because protein binds to the calcium before it can be absorbed. Don't take calcium with iron, caffeine, or excessive salt, because they also decrease absorption or speed excretion. It's best to avoid taking calcium with a big salad because the oxalates in leafy green vegetables combine with calcium to make an insoluble compound, rendering the calcium useless to you. The best time to take calcium supplements that are not in the calcium carbonate form is before meals or at bedtime, when your stomach is relatively empty and absorption will not be influenced by foods, vitamins, or supplements.

The best time to take calcium supplements that are not in calcium carbonate form is before meals or at bedtime.

If you are taking a medication such as Prilosec (omeprazole), its intended effect to reduce stomach acid production will interfere with your ability to absorb calcium carbonate, which should be taken when your stomach is most acidic (usually right after a meal). It's important to take your Prilosec or any stomach acid-inhibiting medications at a time other than with calcium carbonate so that you can absorb calcium more efficiently. Some clinicians believe that Prilosec and other medications that prevent acid production keep stomach acid low even following meals, so other forms of calcium might be best if you need these medications.

It sounds like there are a lot of restrictions around when it's best to take calcium. To make it somewhat easier to figure out a schedule, try this: Take all forms of calcium supplements except carbonate before breakfast. Take calcium carbonate after breakfast as long as you don't have caffeine, foods containing excessive salt or iron, or a leafy green salad. If you are dividing up the calcium carbonate supplements (e.g., two tablets in the morning and two at night), you might try taking them after an evening snack when you're less likely to have the foods or substances that interfere with absorption. Other forms of calcium can be taken between meals throughout the day.

50. There's always a lot of emphasis on eating dairy products for calcium. I can't drink milk or eat cheese because I have lactose intolerance. What can I do to get the calcium necessary for my bones?

Lactose intolerance

Occurs when the small intestine does not make enough lactase, the enzyme required to break down the lactose (milk sugar) in milk products before they enter the large intestine; can cause bloating, pain, gas, and diarrhea.

Lactose intolerance is common. In fact, an estimated 25% of the population of the United States has lactose intolerance. White men and women are affected less often than all other minorities, with 90% of Asians being affected with lactose intolerance.

Lactose intolerance occurs when the small intestine does not make enough lactase, the enzyme required to break down the lactose (milk sugar) in milk products before they enter the large intestine. When the undigested milk products enter the large intestine, you can get bloating, pain, gas, and diarrhea. The symptoms usually appear 30 minutes to 2 hours after eating milk products. Some people can tolerate some milk or milk products if they are eaten in small amounts through the day. The form of lactose intolerance that happens at birth is rare but permanent. Adults can acquire lactose intolerance and sometimes, because of an illness, can have lactose intolerance temporarily.

Don't be discouraged. You might be intolerant, but sometimes you can recondition your body by eating very small amounts of foods that contain lactose and slowly increase the amount over time. For example, you might start with one teaspoon of yogurt for a few days, then a tablespoon for a few days, increase that to a quarter cup for a few days, and so on. The key is to have lactose-containing foods as a regular part of your diet. What you are trying to do is to train your small intestine to start making lactase again. This is a good example of a "use it or lose it" phenomenon. Yogurt is the best tolerated milk product and will also provide you with 200 to 300 mg of calcium per 6- to 8-ounce serving. Hard cheeses, such as cheddar, Swiss, and parmesan, also tend to be easier to digest than milk.

If you try this reconditioning program and it doesn't work, you can certainly get calcium from other sources or try over-the-counter tablets that contain lactase, such as Lactaid® tablets, to help with the digestion of milk products. Whatever you do, be sure that you get adequate calcium because in a recent study, lactose intolerance was associated with low bone mass and increased risk of fracture. Table 4 lists foods that are rich in calcium. You will note that there are non-milk products to choose from.

There is some concern among pediatric clinicians that encouraging dairy product intake in children is not necessary. In fact, there is little evidence that intake of dairy products is associated with increased bone density in children. Children (and adults) can get the same amount of calcium that is in 8 ounces of milk if they consume 8 ounces of fortified orange juice, 1½ cups of calcium-fortified cereal, 2 slices of calcium-fortified bread, or ½ cup of tofu (with calcium sulfate).

If you are unable to tolerate any milk products or if you are a strict vegetarian who consumes no dairy products, you should be doubly careful about getting calcium in other foods as well as supplements. Green leafy vegetables do contain calcium, but it is not absorbed as well as the calcium found in milk products, and therefore only very small amounts of calcium actually make it into the bloodstream. You will not be able to determine the amount of elemental calcium you need in supplements based on the formula described in Question 47. Instead, calculating the amount of calcium you need in the form of supplements might vary somewhat unless you are consistent about the kinds of calcium-rich and calcium-fortified foods you eat. Using Table 4, add up the milligrams of calcium typically found in the foods you eat every day. Subtract that number (you will probably have to average several "typical" days) from the amount of calcium required for your age and sex, found in Table 3. The result is the amount of elemental calcium you need in the form of supplements.

51. I've also been told that I must increase my intake of vitamin D. Should I take a separate vitamin D supplement, or can I get enough through eating the right foods?

Calcium alone won't make strong bones. You must also have enough vitamin D, which is an important but somewhat unusual kind of vitamin. First, it's the only vitamin that can be made by your body when you are out in the sun. And second, liver and kidney enzymes convert vitamin D into a hormone (calcitriol) so that it can aid in strengthening bone. Vitamin D also aids in the absorption of calcium from the intestines so that blood levels stay normal. Vitamin D has two roles in bone health: It is a substance that helps maintain healthy calcium levels in the blood, and it also actually helps to make strong bones and teeth.

The amount of vitamin D that you need varies by age. Children and young adults up to age 25 need 400 international units (IU), as do pregnant and lactating women. Adults between the ages of 25 and 50 only need 200 IU. Adults between the ages of 51 and 70 require 400 IU. And if you're over 70, you need 600 IU of vitamin D. Many clinicians now recommend 600–1000 IU for all adults, especially older individuals who are particularly frail.

Most people don't get enough sunlight to produce an adequate amount of vitamin D, and sun exposure is usually discouraged due to the risks of skin cancer. Therefore, you need supplements or fortified foods to meet the RDA for your age group. The best known vitamin D-fortified food is milk, which contains 100 IU per 8 ounces. But margarine, cereals, canned salmon, and orange juice can also be fortified with vitamin D.

It's hard to determine how much sunshine you need to make enough vitamin D.

It's hard to determine how much sunshine you need to make enough vitamin D. Time estimates differ for warm versus cold weather because sun rays in the cold weather aren't strong enough to trigger the body's vitamin D-making mechanism. Older individuals do not absorb sun well enough to make an adequate supply of vitamin D. Dermatologists are getting into the debate about vitamin D deficiency, as they have long been concerned about unprotected sun exposure and its associated risk of skin cancer. If you wear sunblock regularly, as is recommended by most dermatologists, the sunblock will block your body's ability to make vitamin D. If you are a person of color, you may require longer sun exposure, because Black men and women and probably other persons of color tend to produce less vitamin D than do Whites during the same amount of sun exposure. Because determining how much sun exposure is needed to get adequate vitamin D is so unreliable and because unprotected sun exposure remains controversial among members of the scientific community, it really shouldn't be counted toward your total for vitamin D.

As it relates to bones, vitamin D deficiency can cause fractures, leg pain, and deformities such as bowing of the legs. Severe vitamin D deficiency causes rickets in children and osteomalacia (softening of the bones) in adults.

Vitamin D has not only demonstrated its value for bone health, but a new study of 50,000 men showed that higher levels of vitamin D were associated with a 30% decrease in overall cancer risk, not just colon and prostate cancers. Taking vitamin D supplements has been associated with reducing the risk of multiple sclerosis and diabetes. Vitamin D deficiency has been linked to chronic fatigue, poorer cognitive function among older adults, fibromyalgia, and other problems. Also, pre-menopausal women who consume more than 500 IU of vitamin D may reduce their risk of breast cancer.

Vitamin D also benefits muscles. Older people who have higher levels of vitamin D can get up from a chair and walk better, leading researchers to believe that vitamin D can help reduce falls and fractures. So getting the optimal amount of vitamin D is particularly important for those whose fracture risk is increased due to osteopenia or osteoporosis. Some researchers have found that 800 IU of vitamin D provides the maximum amount of benefit in terms of fractures and falls. This dosage is usually prescribed for older frail adults but more and more clinicians are recommending a daily intake of 600 to 1000 IU for all adults.

Vitamin D also benefits muscles.

For those taking long-term steroids or who have glucocorticoid-induced osteoporosis (GIO), it is advisable to take either supplements of 800 IU of vitamin D per day or an activated form of vitamin D called alfacalcidiol (1 microgram/day) or calcitriol (0.5 microgram/day).

For healthy individuals, a multivitamin containing the RDA of vitamin D for your age group should be enough to meet your daily requirement. You should not exceed 2000 IU through diet or supplements per day. The exception to this is once-a-week Fosamax Plus D, a prescription medication for osteoporosis, which also contains 2800 IU of vitamin D. Although you would be taking 2800 IU in 1 day, the dosage is absorbed by your body over the course of 7 days (see Question 56). Be aware that many calcium preparations also contain varying amounts of vitamin D.

Because vitamin D has been associated with several health benefits, many clinicians are now evaluating blood levels of vitamin D to identify people who may not be getting enough of this important vitamin. This is especially important for people at risk for bone loss and those who already have osteoporosis or osteopenia. The total blood level of vitamin D (total serum 25-OHD) includes both vitamin D made in the body and vitamin D absorbed from foods or supplements. Normal levels of total vitamin D in the blood are above 30 ng/mL. If your level is between 20 and 30 ng/mL, this suggests insufficient vitamin D intake, while a level below 20 ng/mL shows vitamin D deficiency. If your level is below 30 ng/mL, your clinician will likely recommend supplements; the specific type and amount depend on how low your blood level is.

52. Folate has also been in the news regarding its role in osteoporosis. What is folate? How much should I take, and why?

Folate

A vitamin needed for new cell development; helps reduce levels of homocysteine, a substance associated with osteoporotic fractures, heart disease, and stroke; also reduces risk of breast and colon cancer; also called folic acid. A vitamin found in fruits, vegetables, and low-fat dairy products.

Folate, also called folic acid, is well known for its role in preventing spinal cord defects in unborn babies. However, folate also has an important function for everyone—it helps create new cells. One of its most important contributions, either in its natural form found in food or in vitamin supplements, is its role in reducing homocysteine levels. High homocysteine levels are associated with an increased risk of heart disease, stroke, and an increased risk of fracture among older individuals with osteoporosis. Since folate lowers your homocysteine levels, your risk of fracture is also lowered. Some recommend lowering your homocysteine levels by eating fruits, vegetables, and low-fat dairy products, rather than high doses of folate.

In people who have had a stroke, the risk of hip fracture is already increased. High homocysteine levels increase the chances of osteoporotic fractures. Taking folate and vitamin B_{12} significantly reduces the risk of hip fractures by lowering homocysteine levels.

Folate's benefits to your health don't stop at bones. Women, particularly younger women, whose intake equals or exceeds the RDA of 400 micrograms of folate per day, reduce their risk of high blood pressure compared to those whose intake is less than 200 micrograms per day.

Getting at least 400 micrograms per day of folate will benefit your bones and your overall health. Most vitamin supplements contain 100% of your RDA of folate. You should not exceed 1000 micrograms. If you do not take a multivitamin, you should be sure to get folate from foods such as spinach, broccoli, chickpeas, black-eyed peas, asparagus, tomato juice, and fortified breads, cereals, and grains (see Questions 47 and 53).

53. I know there are other vitamins and minerals that are important to bone development. Will I get enough of everything if I take a daily vitamin?

There are several other vitamins and minerals that are vital to your bone development. In addition to calcium, vitamin D, and folate, discussed in previous questions, you should be sure to get enough of vitamins A, B_6, C, and K as well as magnesium, manganese, phosphorus, and fluoride. Although vitamin A, sodium, and phosphorus are important to bones, too much of any of them can interfere with bone formation. People were encouraged to drink fewer carbonated beverages because it was believed that they contain too much phosphorus, but, in fact, a 12-ounce can of low-calorie caffeinated soda contains about 50 mg of phosphorus, only 7% of your RDA. Root beer does not contain any phosphorus. Orange juice actually has about as much phosphorus (approximately 5 mg per ounce) as cola does, and calcium-fortified orange juices have as much as five times the phosphorus as cola, but no one has yet raised concern about phosphorus in orange juice. The real problem with drinking excessive amounts of soda is that soda contains many calories with poor nutritional value and often becomes a substitute for milk and other calcium-rich beverages. Vitamin K is part of building healthy bones and has the added bonus of reducing the risk of hip fracture.

Read the label on your daily vitamin supplement, and then compare the listed amounts for the vitamins and minerals necessary for healthy bones with **Table 6** and Table 3 (Question 47). Note the difference in the tables among the amounts of vitamins and minerals. Some are dosed in milligrams (mg), some in international units (IU), and some in micrograms (mcg).

If your chosen vitamin supplement does not have 100% of any of these vitamins and minerals, you should be taking an additional supplement. Although technically you could get what you need from a diet, most people do not calculate the vitamin and mineral content of every food they eat. It's probably more practical to take a daily vitamin supplement. Taking a daily multivitamin supplement has overall health benefits including helping you to lose weight and preventing chronic diseases such as heart disease or colon and breast cancer.

New daily vitamin supplements seem to appear on the market every day. Although the ones labeled "For

Table 6 Vitamins and Minerals for Bone Health

Vitamin or Mineral	Daily Intake Requirements for Most Adults*	Maximum Daily Amount	Food Sources	Special Notes
Vitamin A	Women >19 y: 700 mcg (2333 IU) Men >19 y: 900mcg (3000 IU)	10,000 IU (3000 mcg)	Organ meats (such as liver, giblets), yellow vegetables (such as carrots, sweet potato, squash), spinach, various fortified cereals	Too much vitamin A can damage bone
Vitamin B$_6$	Women and Men, 31–50 y: 1.3 mg Women >50 y: 1.5 mg Men >50 y: 1.7 mg	100 mg	Bananas, watermelon, fish, chicken, soy, meat, and legumes	Helps with bone development by lowering homocysteine levels (high levels of homocysteine are associated with osteoporotic fractures)
Vitamin C	Women >19 y: 75mg (pregnant/lactating women: up to 120 mg depending on age) Men >19 y: 90 mg	2000 mg	Guava, citrus fruits, red sweet pepper, kiwi, green peppers, tomatoes, strawberries, brussels sprouts, cantaloupe	Helps to make collagen to strengthen bone Smokers should add an extra 35 mg/day to RDA

(cont.)

Table 6 Vitamins and Minerals for Bone Health (*cont.*)

Vitamin or Mineral	Daily Intake Requirements for Most Adults*	Maximum Daily Amount	Food Sources	Special Notes
Vitamin D	Women and Men 31–50 y: 200 IU Women and Men 51–70 y: 400 IU Women and Men >71 y: 600 IU Frail older individuals 800 IU	2000 IU	Fatty fish, fortified milk, margarine, and cereals	Helps the body to absorb calcium and phosphorus from intestines Sunlight on bare skin helps body produce vitamin D Vitamin D helps improve balance
Vitamin K	Women >19 y: 90 mcg Men >19 y: 120 mcg	Not known at this time	Eggs, milk, spinach, many leafy green vegetables, broccoli, liver, cabbage	Helps to make osteocalcin for new bone; believed to reduce risk of hip fractures
Folate (folic acid)	Women and Men >14 y: 400 mcg Pregnancy: 400–600 mcg (high-risk pregnancies require higher amount)	1000 mcg	Fortified cereals, broccoli, many green leafy vegetables, legumes	Helps to reduce homocysteine levels (high levels of homocysteine are associated with osteoporotic fractures)

Magnesium	Women >31 y: 320 mg Men >31: 420 mg	350 mg (this applies only to supplements, not to dietary sources of magnesium)	Pumpkin or sunflower seeds, Brazil nuts, 100% bran cereal, halibut, almonds, cashews, broccoli, spinach, peanut butter, whole wheat breads and cereals	Helps to harden bone
Phosphorus	Women and Men >19 y: 700 mg Children 9–13 y, pregnancy, and lactation: 1250 mg	Women and Men 31–70 y: 4000 mg Women and Men >71 y: 3000 mg	Almonds, green peas, eggs, poultry, potatoes, milk and dairy products, meat, fish, broccoli	Helps to harden bone
Manganese	Women >19 y: 1.8 mg Men>19 y: 2.3 mg	11 mg	Whole grains, legumes, nuts, tea	Helps regulate certain enzymes related to bone growth

*Note differences in micrograms (mcg), milligrams (mg), and international units (IU).

Sources: Harvard Medical School. *The Benefits and Risks of Vitamins and Minerals: What You Need to Know.* Boston, MA: Harvard Medical School–Harvard Health Publications; 2003.

Fact Sheets, Office of Dietary Supplements, National Institutes of Health. Available at: http://dietary-supplements.info.nih.gov/. Accessed August 2005.

and U.S. Department of Health and Human Services. *Bone Health and Osteoporosis: A Report of the Surgeon General.* Rockville, MD: U.S. Department of Health and Human Services, Office of the Surgeon General; 2004.

Bone Health" logically would contain the adequate types and amounts of the vitamins and minerals that you need to maintain healthy bones, this may not be true. For example, different age groups need different amounts of vitamins and minerals. Read labels carefully. The products may also contain substances you don't need at all. For example, men and postmenopausal women usually don't need to take iron because they don't have menstrual periods to lower their iron levels, and they get enough iron in their daily intake of food.

54. What are isoflavones? Are they effective for treating osteoporosis?

Isoflavones are **phytoestrogens**, weak estrogenic substances found in plants. Isoflavones are most notably found in soy and red clover. The isoflavones that are found in soy are different from the isoflavones found in red clover. Sometimes manufacturers mix the different isoflavones into one product. For example, Rimostil® is a blend of isoflavones derived from red clover, while Estroven contains 55 mg of isoflavones derived from soy and another plant extract. Most isoflavone products are available over the counter and are not held to the same Food and Drug Administration (FDA) regulations as prescription medications. One isoflavone product, Fosteum®, meets the FDA GRAS standard, meaning "generally regarded as safe," and is available by prescription as a medical food. Fosteum contains a combination of genistein (isoflavone purified from soy), zinc, and vitamin D. It has been shown to improve BMD, but fracture data are not available (see Table 7).

Manufacturers extract isoflavones from soy protein and red clover, but isoflavones are also found in foods such as soy products and other legumes such as chickpeas.

Isoflavone

A type of phytoestrogen found most notably in soy and red clover.

Phytoestrogens

Weak, estrogen-like substances that are in plants. Can be eaten in whole foods, such as soy, or extracted from red clover in the form of isoflavones and made into supplements.

When you eat foods containing isoflavones, your intestines convert the plant chemicals into estrogen-like substances that are absorbed into the circulation and can then bind with estrogen receptors, making them act like estrogen in some ways. And we know that estrogen is a major component in building and maintaining strong bones, particularly in women, which is why there is such interest in the potential role of isoflavones and phyto-estrogens in the prevention and treatment of bone loss.

Because isoflavones have been found to act like estrogen in the body, isoflavones are being studied not only for their effects on the hot flashes associated with menopause, but also for their effects on bone health. Several small studies have shown some promise in reducing bone loss and increasing bone mineral density without some of the side effects of estrogen observed in other scientific studies. For example, isoflavones don't seem to increase breast density, increase endometrial thickness, or exert the same negative effects on your heart health. Further study is needed to confirm the bone findings reported when isoflavone supplements are taken. Isoflavones are considered safe when taken with other medications, such as the prescription medications described in Questions 55 to 67.

Some people choose to eat soy instead of taking soy isoflavone supplements. The FDA has approved product labeling that says, "Diets low in saturated fat and cholesterol that include 25 grams of soy protein a day may reduce the risk of heart disease." One serving of soy protein burger (for example) provides 9 grams of soy protein. In order to use this claim on labeling, a soy product must be low in fat, cholesterol, and sodium and contain at least 6.25 grams of soy protein. But it's not clear how many milligrams of isoflavones are in each gram of soy protein. The degree to which you absorb isoflavones from soy will depend on the food product and the bacteria in your intestines. An 8-ounce glass of soy milk, when converted in your intestines, can provide 20 to 45 mg of isoflavones. There's no firm evidence at this time that eating soy or taking soy supplements will improve your bone density; however, eating soy is still a good strategy as part of a healthy diet, and many soy foods, like tofu, are a good source of calcium. Question 71 discusses other complementary and alternative therapies for osteoporosis, and Question 99 discusses future developments, including a synthetic isoflavone that is being researched for its effects on bone.

55. Who should be treated for bone loss? What is the FRAX® algorithm and how is it used? What types of medications are usually prescribed for osteoporosis and osteopenia?

If you are told you have osteopenia or are diagnosed with osteoporosis, calcium and vitamin D supplementation with appropriate exercise may not be enough to decrease bone loss or to build bone. You may need a prescription medication. Some medications are only prescribed for women, and others are prescribed for both women and men.

If your T-score is in the osteoporosis range, your clinician will likely recommend medication in addition to lifestyle changes such as exercise and adequate intake of calcium and vitamin D. Most clinicians also agree that if your T-score is in the osteopenia range of −2.0 or lower or if your T-score is −1.0 to −2.5 and you have also had a low-trauma fracture, you should be treated with medication and lifestyle changes. However, consensus has been lacking about whether to start medication therapy for individuals with T-scores in the −1 to −2 range or when risk factors other than low-trauma fracture are present.

The World Health Organization (WHO) recognized the lack of consensus about treatment for people with low bone mass (T-score −1.0 to −2.5). To assist with determining who might benefit from starting medication therapy, the WHO developed the Fracture Risk Assessment Tool (FRAX®) algorithm to identify the 10-year probability for having a hip fracture or major osteoporotic fracture (i.e., spine, hip, forearm, or humerus [upper arm bone]).

The algorithm is available online (www.shef.ac.uk/ FRAX/), and users can identify a specific country and language. United States users specify among four different ethnic/racial groups: Caucasian, Black, Hispanic, or Asian. Risk factor information is entered for 11 different risks (see **Box 1**) and the femoral neck raw BMD value in g/cm^2 (or the total hip can be substituted if the femoral neck is not known; other site

---

| BOX 1 | *Risk Factors Used for the WHO FRAX Online Algorithm* |

- Age and date of birth
- Cigarette smoking status (yes/no)
- Femoral neck BMD score in g/cm^2; specify DXA or other type of measure
- If parent ever had a hip fracture (yes/no)
- If three or more units of alcohol are consumed per day (yes/no)
- If patient has history of prior fracture (yes/no)

(continued)

> ### BOX 1   *(Continued)*
>
> - Patient's height in centimeters
> - Patient's weight in kilograms
> - Presence of rheumatoid arthritis (yes/no)
> - Presence of secondary osteoporosis (yes/no)
> - Sex (male/female)
> - Use of glucocorticoid medications (yes/no)

BMD values cannot be used because the tool has not been tested using values from other sites).

The FRAX algorithm is user-friendly. Position your computer cursor over the "Calculation Tool" area on the top banner, move down to click on the United States country group, and select the appropriate ethnic/racial subgroup. Next enter the appropriate values for each of the 11 risk factors and your raw hip BMD value in g/cm^2. Specify if the test was a DXA or other type, then click on "Calculate" to identify your personal 10-year risk for hip or major osteoporotic fracture. Height and weight must be entered as centimeters and kilograms. The FRAX site provides a conversion tool from inches to centimeters and pounds to kilograms on the same Web page, located on the far left of the computer screen (see **Figure 11**).

The FRAX results are intended to assist with clinical decision making and do not provide a definitive result for clinicians to follow. The tool uses several risk factors that are known to be important for bone health (see Box 1), but other factors are also important. Additionally, some of the factors that are included are entered simply as *yes* or *no* responses when in reality the amount is important. For example, long-term

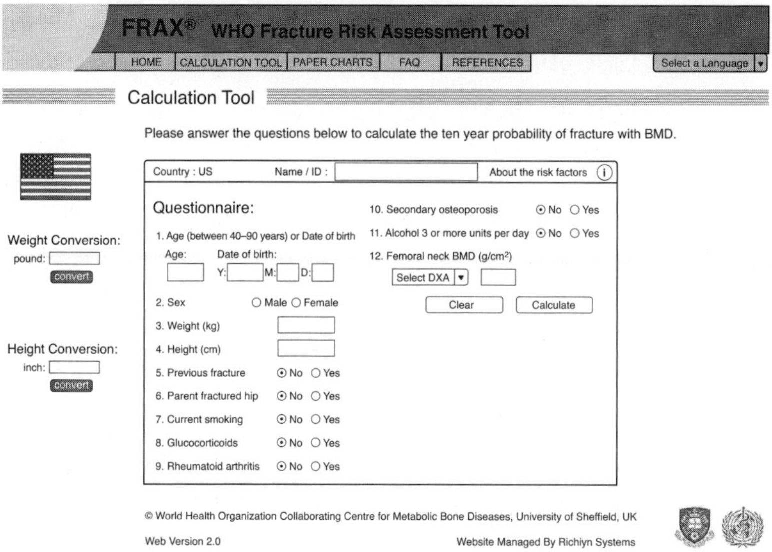

Figure 11 FRAX® algorithm.
Source: Image used with permission of the WHO Collaborating Centre for Metabolic Bone Diseases, University of Sheffield. FRAX® is registered to Professor JA Kanis, University of Sheffield.

steroid use is entered as *yes* or *no*, but in clinical practice it is known that higher doses of steroids have greater effects on bone than do lower doses.

The FRAX algorithm is used by clinicians to identify who might benefit from starting medication therapy for bone loss, and it is specifically intended for patients whose BMD levels fall in the low bone mass category (−1.0 to −2.5) and who have not used medication previously. The current version of the FRAX is in a test, or "beta," format and will be changed in the future after it has been used clinically and problems or necessary changes are identified. For the present, it is a very useful tool for assisting with clinical decisions about who might benefit from using medication. FRAX results are expected to be included in BMD test reports to clinicians by the end of 2009 (see Question 33). Studies have determined what thresholds of the FRAX

121

results for both hip and major osteoporotic fracture are cost-effective on a population basis for starting medication treatment.

Based on this information, the National Osteoporosis Foundation (NOF) set clinical recommendations for starting medication if you are a postmenopausal woman or a man over 50 if you have:

- A BMD T-score at the total hip, femoral neck, or spine of −2.5 or lower and no other causes of bone loss ("secondary osteoporosis")
- Fracture(s) at the spine (either identified on x-rays or other tests or by clinical examination) or at the hip
- Previous fracture(s) at other sites together with low bone mass (T-score of −1.0 to −2.5) at the hip or spine
- Low bone mass (T-score of −1.0 to −2.5) at the spine or hip together with secondary causes that are associated with high risks for fracture (e.g., use of glucocorticoids, immobilization)
- Low bone mass (T-score of −1.0 to −2.5) at the spine or hip together with a FRAX calculated 10-year fracture probability at the hip of 3% or higher or for any major osteoporotic fracture of 20% or higher

The types of prescription medication used fall into two categories. The first category of medications is called **antiresorptive agents**. They are intended to work on the osteoclasts to inhibit bone resorption, meaning that the medications interfere with the cells that are trying to break down old bone. Estrogen therapy (ET) is one of these types of medications and for postmenopausal women has been found to be very effective in the prevention of osteoporosis. ET is appropriate for preventing osteoporosis in postmenopausal women who are experiencing significant menopausal symptoms (see

Antiresorptive agents

Medications and substances that decrease bone resorption (bone breakdown).

Questions 64–66). Other medications that fall into the group of drugs intended to prevent further loss by slowing down the breakdown of bone include **bisphosphonates**, calcitonin, and **estrogen agonists/antagonists** (which used to be known as selective estrogen receptor modulators [SERMs] until September 2007 when the FDA changed the terminology). Questions 56 to 65 contain a full discussion of each drug. Although the medications do not make new bone directly, they do assist in increasing bone density by slowing down the rate at which old bone is broken down. In each question, specific information about the bisphosphonate medications are presented. It is important to note that a recent study identified that all of the bisphosphonates are basically equally beneficial in treating bone loss. Some differences in specific studies may have been caused by the numbers of patients who participated, time for the study overall, how data were collected or reported, and so forth. In the end, bisphosphonates, as well as the other treatment choices for bone loss, are extremely effective options. Discussing the various possibilities with your clinician and taking into account what will fit into your life, such as a daily versus monthly pill, an intravenous infusion, or a subcutaneous injection, are very important, as staying on the medication is what relates most strongly to how well it works.

There currently is only one FDA-approved medication in the second category of medications used to treat osteoporosis. This medication is called an **anabolic agent**, which works with osteoblasts to actually build bone (see Question 62).

The most important thing for you to remember is that prescription medications do not usually contain calcium or vitamin D; however, Fosamax (alendronate) Plus D does contain vitamin D and Actonel (risedronate)

Bisphosphonates

A group of antiresorptive agents, such as Fosamax, Boniva, and Actonel, which slow the rate at which bone is broken down.

Estrogen agonist/ antagonist

Antiresorptive medications such as Evista that help to reduce bone loss by their positive estrogenic effects.

Anabolic agent

Medication, steroid hormone, or substance intended to build bone; examples are Forteo (teriperatide) and testosterone.

Lifestyle Changes and Treatments

with Calcium does contain calcium. Fosamax Plus D contains 2800 IU of vitamin D, a week's worth of vitamin D. Actonel with Calcium is a new way of packaging the once-weekly Actonel dose. The package includes 4 weeks of medication. Each week has one 35-mg Actonel tablet and six 1250-mg calcium carbonate tablets (500 mg elemental calcium each) to take on the days that Actonel is not taken. Even if you take the prescription medication faithfully, you will not get the full benefit of its effects without getting adequate calcium and vitamin D in your diet or by supplements. So, make sure that your prescription medication has a chance to work by remembering to take the necessary amount of calcium and vitamin D. If you are prescribed a bisphosphonate, you must NOT take calcium and the medication at the same time. Bisphosphonates must be taken alone, on an empty stomach, with a plain glass of water first thing in the morning or when you are up for the rest of the day. You must not lie down or eat or drink anything else for 30–60 minutes, depending on the specific medicine. You must take your calcium later. Further instructions on how to take bisphosphonates appear in Questions 56 to 60.

Bisphosphonates must be taken alone, on an empty stomach, with a plain glass of water first thing in the morning or when you are up for the rest of the day.

Adherence with taking any medication prescribed for you is very important. A recent study showed that the majority of women stop taking their prescribed bisphosphonate medication before 1 year is up and, although weekly dosing was better than daily dosing, many on weekly dosing still did not stick to their medication regimen. The researchers speculate that there are two reasons why women don't stay on their bisphosphonate medication regimens. First, osteoporosis is a chronic disease, but you can't see it or feel it unless you fracture a bone, so it may be difficult to justify the expense for medications and establish the ongoing routine for taking them. Secondly, because it is necessary to follow strict guidelines when taking the medication either daily or weekly, sticking to the regimen can be trying. The obvious downside to not taking your medication regularly, whether it's a bisphosphonate or something else, is that you will not benefit from its intended effects. You will not improve your bone mineral density and your fracture risk will continue to increase (see **Table 7**).

Table 7 Summary of Prescription Products for Osteopenia and Osteoporosis

Class of Products[*]	Clinical Uses	Considerations
Bisphosphonates (Actonel, Boniva, Fosamax, Reclast)[†]	Osteoporosis prevention and treatment	• Caution if allergic; upper gastrointestinal disease (e.g., ulcers or reflux) or kidney disease • Take tablet by mouth first thing in the morning on an empty stomach with a full glass of water, remain upright and take no other food or drink for at least 30 minutes to 1 hour depending on which bisphosphonate • Dosing schedules are dependent on the products (some tablets can be taken daily, once per week, or once per month; IV therapies are once every 6 or 12 months) • Do not take antacids/calcium until 2 hours after taking oral bisphosphonates • Oral bisphosphonates may cause inflammation of stomach or esophagus; nausea; vomiting; constipation; diarrhea; flatulence; ulcer; swelling; abdominal, muscle, back, or joint pain; or (rarely) osteonecrosis of the jaw after dental surgery • Bisphosphonates are not a substitute for calcium and vitamin D; both are critical to successful treatment with bisphosphonates • IV forms usually require office visit for administration

(cont.)

Table 7   Summary of Prescription Products for Osteopenia and Osteoporosis (*cont.*)

Class of Products*	Clinical Uses	Considerations
Calcitonin (Miacalcin NS, Fortical)†	Osteoporosis and vertebral fractures	• Administered as a nasal spray • Has pain-relieving effect on fractures due to osteoporosis • Caution if allergic • May cause spasms of large airways, nausea, vomiting, flushing, rash, itching, warmth, nighttime urination, eye pain, reduced appetite, swelling, abdominal pain, salty taste
Estrogen therapies‡ (e.g., Activella, Alora, Climara, Estrace, Estraderm, FemHRT, Menest, Premarin, Vivelle-Dot, others)†	Prevention of osteoporosis (for women only)	• Should be prescribed for prevention of osteoporosis only if moderate-to-severe hot flashes and night sweats are present • Also effective in alleviating most symptoms of menopause • Improves balance and reduces falls • Comes in several forms (i.e., pills, patch, ring, cream, spray, gel) • May cause vaginal bleeding/spotting; breast changes/tenderness; bloating/cramps; weight changes; nausea; vomiting; headache; swelling; elevated blood pressure; hair changes; rash; vaginal yeast infections; vision changes; difficulty wearing contact lenses; and, rarely, depression; uterine fibroid growth; worsening of asthma; blood clots; stroke; heart attack; dementia; cancers of the breast, ovaries, or uterine lining; problems with gallbladder, liver, or pancreas • May not be used in combination with Evista (one combination of an estrogen agonist/antagoist with estrogen is currently being investigated)

(cont.)

Table 7 Summary of Prescription Products for Osteopenia and Osteoporosis (*cont.*)

Class of Products*	Clinical Uses	Considerations
Low-dose estrogen patch (Menostar)†	Prevention of osteoporosis (for women only)	• Very low-dose estrogen patch specifically tested and pre-scribed for preventing osteo-porosis, also provides relief for hot flashes • All contraindications and side effects of estrogen apply to use of medication • May not be used in combination with Evista or other estrogen therapies • Does not improve BMD as much as higher-dose estrogen products
Raloxifene (Evista)†	Prevention and treatment of osteoporosis (for women only)	• Only estrogen agonist/antagonist available for osteoporosis prevention and treatment • Cannot be taken with MHT (menopause hormone therapy) • Caution if allergy, blood clots, high triglyceride levels, using hormone therapy • May cause hot flashes, infection, flu-like symptoms, joint pain, sinusitis, nausea, weight gain, inflammation of mouth/throat, depression, cough, leg cramps, rash, insomnia, stomach upset, or clots
Teriparitide (Forteo)†	Osteoporosis treatment	• Only FDA-approved anabolic (bone-building) medication • Given by daily injection at home • Usually used only if other treat-ments are ineffective or not tolerated • Caution if allergy, bone cancer, history of radiation to bone, uri-nary stones, parathyroid disease, bone disease • May cause low blood pressure, dizziness, weakness, joint pain, leg cramps, fainting, chest pain

(cont.)

Table 7 Summary of Prescription Products for Osteopenia and Osteoporosis (*cont.*)

Class of Products*	Clinical Uses	Considerations
Genestein + citrated zinc + cholecalciferol (Fosteum Rx®)§	Prevention of osteoporosis	• Prescription medical food • Meets FDA standards for "generally recognized as safe" (GRAS) • Not recommended if taking estrogen or hormone therapy or estrogen agonist/antagonist • May cause breast tenderness, nausea, constipation, abdominal pain • Contraindication/caution if pregnant, nursing, breast/estrogen-dependent cancer

Note: All medications have associated benefits, risks, and side effects. These should be discussed with your clinician before starting any medication.

*Prescription medications are not a substitute for taking calcium and vitamin D. You must take the appropriate amount of calcium and vitamin D regardless of medication regimen (see Tables 3 and 6).

†See individual tables for Actonel (Table 9), Boniva (Table 10), Fosamax (Table 8), Reclast (Table 11), Evista (Table 13), Forteo (Table 14), Menostar (Table 16), Miacalcin NS/Fortical (Table 15), and estrogen therapies (Table 17).

‡Some estrogen products listed contain progestin as well as estrogen.

§A prescription medical food

Certain groups of people should receive prescription medications for the prevention and treatment of osteoporosis. According to the American College of Rheumatology, bisphosphonates (see Questions 56–58) should be prescribed to the following groups who are receiving glucocorticoid therapy (such as for rheumatoid arthritis, asthma, inflammatory bowel disease, or lupus):

• To prevent bone loss in individuals in whom long-term glucocorticoid (steroid) treatment (doses of 5 mg or more per day) has been initiated
• Patients who already have GIO with documented low bone mineral density or recent fracture
• Patients receiving glucocorticoids who have sustained fractures while on estrogen therapy or in whom estrogen therapy has not been well tolerated.

56. I was prescribed Fosamax (alendronate). What is that? What are the contraindications to taking it, and are there any side effects? I've heard that Fosamax can be very tough on the stomach. Is that true?

Fosamax (alendronate) is one of the bisphosphonates, a group of drugs used to treat or prevent osteoporosis as well as to prevent bone loss in early postmenopausal women. Fosamax does this by decreasing bone turnover. Fosamax and the three other FDA-approved bisphosphonates for treating or preventing osteoporosis—Actonel (risedronate), Boniva® (ibandronate), and Reclast® (zoledronic acid)—don't actually build bone, but they are very effective in preventing further breakdown of bone. By slowing bone turnover, bone mineral density increases. In fact, bisphosphonates can decrease spinal fracture risk in as little as 1 year of treatment. A fifth bisphosphonate, Didronel® (etidronate), also affects bone turnover and is FDA-approved for the treatment of Paget's disease. Questions 57 to 60 discuss Actonel, Boniva, Reclast, and Didronel.

Fosamax is FDA-approved for prescription daily or once a week in different doses for the purposes of preventing or treating osteoporosis in postmenopausal women, treating to increase bone mass in men with osteoporosis, or treating glucocorticoid-induced osteoporosis (GIO) in men or women with low BMD who are receiving daily doses of glucocorticoids ≥ 7.5 mg. The dosage of Fosamax for GIO is one 5-mg tablet by mouth per day for men and women or 10 mg per day for postmenopausal women who are not taking estrogen. The BMD in individuals with GIO significantly increases after about 1 year of treatment using Fosamax. Either the 5-mg per day dose or one 35-mg tablet by mouth once a week is used to treat postmenopausal women with osteopenia, because the goal of osteopenia treatment is osteoporosis prevention. For the treatment of osteoporosis in postmenopausal women or to increase bone mass in men with osteoporosis, the dosage is one 10-mg tablet per day or one 70-mg tablet once a week. A month's supply of tablets, whether taken daily or weekly, costs about $85 to $90 without insurance coverage or co-pays.

Results of a 6-year study showed that women taking Fosamax and women taking EPT (estrogen-progestin therapy) both had increases in BMD. Fosamax and EPT were discontinued after 4 years and once again, BMD decreased in all of the postmenopausal women. However, those who had taken Fosamax had less bone loss after 2 years than those who took EPT.

Yes, it's true that Fosamax can be tough on your stomach, and if you already have stomach ulcers or reflux disease, it should be used with extreme caution. Stomach upset and the risk for ulcers is further increased if you are taking nonsteroidal anti-inflammatory medications (NSAIDs) such as ibuprofen (e.g., Motrin, Nuprin), naproxen (e.g., Aleve), or aspirin while you are on Fosamax. You can minimize the negative effects such as heartburn and stomach upset by following strict guidelines. Whether you take Fosamax daily or weekly, you must take it using these same guidelines:

• If you are on the weekly version of Fosamax, pick a day and stick with it. Most people pick Sunday unless they are too tempted to go back to sleep.

Fosamax tablets come with tiny stickers to put on your calendar as reminders to take it. If you happen to forget to take it on the day it is due (e.g., Sunday), then take it the very next day (e.g., Monday).

- Take it on an empty stomach. Food interferes with its absorption. So does any liquid except PLAIN water.
- You must swallow the tablet whole. Do not chew or suck on it.
- When you are up for the day (meaning that you are not going to lie down after taking it), take the tablet with a 6- to 8-ounce glass of PLAIN water, not seltzer water, not fruit-flavored water, and not any other beverage made with water. Never take Fosamax before retiring for the night. Only take it with plain water.
- Take nothing else for at least 30 minutes. Do not take calcium, vitamin D, minerals, or antacids within 2 hours of taking Fosamax.
- Do not lie down or bend at the waist. Don't go back to bed. Bending at the waist or lying down can make the medication reflux into your esophagus and increase the chance of heartburn.
- You may eat and take other medications after 30 minutes, except milk and those items previously mentioned.

Bisphosphonates may cause inflammation of the stomach or esophagus, nausea, vomiting, constipation, diarrhea, flatulence, ulcer, swelling, or abdominal, muscle, back, or joint pain. Although very rare, **osteonecrosis of the jaw** (ONJ; deterioration of bone tissue) following dental surgery has been reported in patients taking long-term intravenous bisphosphonate therapy used for treating cancer and reducing bone pain and cancer-related high levels of blood calcium. Most reports were in patients taking intravenous (IV) bisphosphonate therapy. Extremely rare cases have been reported in those taking the medications by mouth.

Osteonecrosis of the jaw

Deterioration of jaw bone associated with tooth loss, local infection, and delayed healing; leads to death of local jaw bone tissue.

ONJ happens when bone tissue in the jaw is exposed for 3 months or more and nonhealing lesions are identified. Patients at risk are people with cancer who are taking high-dose IV bisphosphonates, have poor dental health, have abnormalities in the mouth bones, have injuries to their gums, or are taking medications that interfere with healing. ONJ is very rare, affecting 2% to 10% of patients taking high-dose IV bisphos-phonates for bone-related cancers. Occurrence rates among healthy people taking bisphosphonates for osteoporosis prevention or treatment are estimated at less than 1% (0.001% to 0.002%). ONJ is most likely to happen after an invasive dental procedure. It is important to inform your dentist if you are taking or have previously taken bisphosphonates and to main-tain good dental hygiene (brushing regularly, having regular dental check-ups and cleanings, avoiding sticky candies, and using fluoride toothpaste), which can further reduce the small risk for ONJ.

Fosamax is strictly contraindicated if you have an allergy to bisphosphonates or advanced kidney disease. Caution should be used when Fosamax is taken by anyone with existing stomach or intestinal disease. **Table 8** summarizes the contraindications and consid-erations for taking Fosamax. While the majority of Fosamax's side effects are related to heartburn, you should always immediately report chest pain, difficulty swallowing, or severe midline heartburn.

The FDA also approved Fosamax Plus D™, a weekly tablet that contains the same 70 mg of alendronate found in the weekly Fosamax tablet, but also has added vitamin D. The 2800 IU of vitamin D in Fosamax Plus D is the typical weekly amount recommended for peo-ple aged 51 to 70. If you are over the age of 70, you will

Table 8 Fosamax (alendronate)

Trade Name (Generic Name) [Manufacturer] How Supplied	Clinical Uses	Contraindications	Most Common Side Effects and Adverse Reactions	Special Considerations
Fosamax, Fosamax Plus D (alendronate) [Merck] 5, 10, 35, 40, 70 mg tablets as Fosamax 70 mg tablet as Fosamax Plus D (2800 IU Vitamin D)	Postmenopausal women at risk for developing osteoporosis Postmenopausal women or men who have osteoporosis Men and women who are taking ≥ 7.5 mg of glucocorticoids daily and who have low bone density Paget's disease in men and women	Allergy to bisphosphonates Esophageal abnormalities Low blood calcium Poor kidney function Inability to remain upright for 30 minutes	GI: acid reflux, nausea, vomiting, diarrhea, abdominal pain, flatulence, esophageal ulcer Bone or muscle pain Get immediate help for difficulty swallowing, midline chest pain, severe vomiting, or severe abdominal pain	Take first thing after rising for the day on an empty stomach with a full glass of plain water; remain upright and take no other food or drink for at least 30 minutes Can be taken weekly in some instances Use caution if upper gastrointestinal disease (e.g., ulcers or reflux) or kidney disease Found to be safe up to 10 years of use Do not take calcium, other minerals, or milk products within 2 hours of taking Fosamax Compliance with medication schedule important to increasing BMD Fosamax Plus D contains 2800 IU of vitamin D, a week's worth of vitamin D for individuals aged 51 to 70 If prescribed by a specialist for women of childbearing age, they must be on an effective method of birth control and counseled about the unknown long-term effects on future pregnancy If you are taking Fosamax Plus D, it may still be necessary to take a daily supplement of vitamin D (see Table 3 for the RDA for your age) RDA of calcium and vitamin D are also important for increasing BMD; both are needed on the day Fosamax is taken (at least 2 hours after Fosamax) In very rare cases could increase the risk for osteonecrosis of the jaw following dental surgery

need to make sure that you still get an additional 200 IU per day of vitamin D. Table 8 reviews the indications and considerations for using Fosamax.

The long-term safety of Fosamax has been established in those taking it for 10 years or more. Several studies have shown that bone density does increase, and safety is maintained in patients who take Fosamax for ≥10 years. Additionally, some bone protection persists even after Fosamax is stopped in those who have taken it for 5 years continuously. Very long-term use of Fosamax may be associated with oversuppression of bone turnover. This causes the quality of the bone to suffer because there is not the usual turnover of older bone tissue due to the inhibition of osteoclast activity, rendering the bone more fragile. One study found that longer use of Fosamax was associated with higher risk for low-trauma fracture of the thigh bone (femur). More research is needed to identify whether this increased risk for fracture is only related to long-term use of alendronate or to all bisphosphonates.

Half-life

Time it takes the body to metabolize or inactivate half of the amount of a medication that was taken.

The long-term effects of Fosamax could be a concern even after it is discontinued. The **half-life** of Fosamax can exceed 10 years. This means that it can take a very long time for the body to eliminate all of the Fosamax that has been absorbed. Effects on bone are likely to be positive, but it is not clear how a future pregnancy would be affected by the continued effects of Fosamax or other bisphosphonates. Fosamax is not FDA-approved for use in premenopausal women except those with GIO. If a premenopausal woman had a fragility fracture (see Question 74), a specialist may consider treatment with a bisphosphonate. This would only be considered if other potential causes for the fracture were ruled out and if she were on a very reliable method of birth control or unable to conceive.

57. What is Actonel (risedronate)? Is it like Fosamax (alendronate)?

Actonel (risedronate) is another bisphosphonate prescribed to reduce bone turnover to treat or prevent osteoporosis. It can be taken as 5 mg daily, 35 mg weekly, 75 mg on 2 consecutive days once monthly, or as 150 mg on a single day once a month by mouth. Like other bisphosphonates, you must be conscientious about following the guidelines listed in Question 57 for taking Fosamax or any bisphosphonate medication. You must take Actonel with PLAIN water on an empty stomach and remain upright (sitting or standing) for 30 minutes. Actonel must be taken prior to the first beverage or food of the day. In other words, nothing should be consumed for 30 minutes after taking Actonel with plain water. Flex dosing (taking Actonel 2 hours after food or beverage and at least 2 hours prior to consuming more food or beverage) is approved in other countries but was not approved by the FDA in the United States because it has the potential to reduce the absorption of the medicine. Do not take calcium and other minerals or milk within 2 hours of taking Actonel.

The FDA also approved new packaging of weekly Actonel called Actonel with Calcium. This packaging includes a month's supply of medication. There are four packets, one for each week, containing seven pills—one 35 mg tablet of Actonel and six 1250 mg tablets of calcium carbonate (500 mg of elemental calcium). The manufacturer developed this packaging for individuals taking weekly Actonel to assist them in remembering to take calcium. The directions say to take Actonel 1 day according to the guidelines described above and to take one calcium tablet with food on each of the other 6 days of the week. Remember that you must also get adequate vitamin D so that the calcium is absorbed. On the day you take the Actonel tablet, it is still important to get your RDA of calcium, but you must not take calcium supplements within 2 hours after taking the Actonel tablet. The 500 mg of elemental calcium carbonate supplied in the daily calcium tablet that comes in the Actonel with Calcium package may not be enough to meet your RDA for calcium, so you may need additional calcium supplements.

Actonel is FDA-approved for the treatment or prevention of postmenopausal osteoporosis in women. It is also approved for the treatment and prevention of glucocorticoid-induced osteoporosis (GIO) in adults who are initiating or continuing oral glucorcorticoid medications at doses of ≥7.5 mg daily. Actonel has also been approved for the treatment of Paget's disease (see Question 60).

In a recent study that compared the effect of weekly Fosamax on bone mineral density with the effect of weekly Actonel on bone mineral density, Fosamax showed a greater increase in BMD and a greater decrease in bone turnover. But those taking Actonel had fewer fractures than those taking Fosamax. We already know that both Fosamax and Actonel are effective in reducing fracture risk, which is, after all, the point of treating osteoporosis. However, the increase in bone density did not have the expected level of reducing fracture risk in those taking Fosamax. Although Actonel users reported slightly fewer stomach and intestinal (GI) complaints, there was essentially no difference between the GI effects of Actonel and Fosamax.

This study illustrates how important it is for you to work with your clinician to find the best medication for you. For example, both medications, weekly Fosamax and weekly Actonel, are effective in decreasing bone turnover, increasing bone mineral density, and reducing fracture risk significantly more than taking a **placebo**, based on many years of clinical trials. But sometimes people tolerate one medication better than another. And sometimes clinicians feel more strongly about the success of one medication over another. You may even be influenced by friends who have taken medication for bone loss and experienced side effects less frequently with one medication over another. The cost of Actonel and Fosamax are about the same. But remember that each person's medical history and bones are different. You and your clinician should make your decision together, whether you choose a bisphosphonate or not.

Placebo

An inactive substance that contains no medication or active ingredient; to be given to participants in a clinical trial to determine the effectiveness of a specific treatment or medication.

Like Fosamax, most side effects of Actonel are related to the esophagus (usually causing heartburn), but if you are taking one of these drugs it is important to report chest pain, difficulty swallowing, or severe midline heartburn immediately. If you are taking NSAIDs such as ibuprofen, aspirin, or naproxen for pain management—which are known to increase the risk of developing acid stomach or ulcers—together with a bisphosphonate, the risk for gastrointestinal effects can be increased further. **Table 9** summarizes information about Actonel.

Also like Fosamax, the long-term effects of Actonel could be a concern after it is discontinued. Although the half-life of Actonel is measured in days instead of years as in the case of Fosamax, it is not clear how a future pregnancy would be affected by the continued effects of Actonel or other bisphosphonates. Actonel is not FDA approved for use in premenopausal women

137

Table 9   Actonel (risedronate) and Actonel with Calcium

Trade Name (Generic Name) [Manufacturer] How Supplied	Clinical Uses	Contraindications	Most Common Side Effects and Adverse Reactions	Special Considerations
Actonel (risedronate) [Procter & Gamble Pharmaceuticals] 5, 30, 35, 75, 150 mg tablets Actonel with Calcium (risedronate with calcium carbonate) [The Alliance for Better Bone Health, a collaboration between Procter & Gamble Pharmaceuticals and Aventis Pharmaceuticals] 35 mg risedronate packaged with six calcium carbonate tablets, each 1250 mg	Prevention and treatment of postmenopausal osteoporosis Treatment of glucocorticoid-induced osteoporosis Prevention of osteoporosis in people taking ≥ 7.5 mg of glucocorticoids daily Paget's disease	Allergy to bisphosphonates Esophageal abnormalities Low blood calcium Poor kidney function Inability to remain upright (sitting or standing) for 30 minutes	GI: acid reflux, nausea, vomiting, diarrhea, abdominal pain, flatulence, esophageal ulcer Bone or muscle pain Get immediate help for difficulty swallowing, midline chest pain, or severe abdominal pain	Take first thing after rising for the day on an empty stomach with a full glass of plain water, remain upright and take no other food or drink for at least 30 minutes Can be taken weekly or monthly (5 mg, 35 mg), monthly on 2 consecutive days (75 mg), or monthly as a single dose taken 1 day each month (150 mg) Use caution if upper gastrointestinal disease (e.g., ulcers or reflux) or kidney disease Do not take calcium, other minerals, or milk products within 2 hours of taking Actonel Adherence to medication schedule important for increasing BMD RDA of calcium and vitamin D are also important for increasing BMD; both are needed on the day Actonel is taken (at least 2 hours after Actonel) If prescribed by a specialist for women of child-bearing age, they must be on an effective method of birth control and counseled about the unknown long-term effects on future pregnancy In very rare cases could increase the risk for osteonecrosis of the jaw following dental surgery

except those with GIO. If a premenopausal woman had a fragility fracture (see Question 74), a specialist may consider treatment with a bisphosphonate. This would only be considered if other potential causes for the fracture were ruled out and if she were on a very reliable method of birth control or unable to conceive.

58. What is Boniva (ibandronate)? Is it also called Bonviva?

Boniva is approved for once-a-month oral dosing by the FDA. It was the first bisphosphonate available for monthly administration. Boniva is available in the United States and is also marketed in other countries under the brand name Bonviva. Boniva is approved for the prevention and treatment of postmenopausal osteoporosis and is available as a 2.5-mg tablet taken daily, 150-mg tablet taken monthly, or intravenous injection given in a 3-mg dose every 3 months. The daily dose is available in the United States on a limited basis because the monthly dose is more effective and it is easier to remember a monthly pill. The intravenous dose is administered in a clinical office and takes only a few minutes.

All dosages tested in multiple research studies increased BMD at the lumbar spine and other bones, and fractures were significantly reduced at the spine. Although the very long-term effects of Boniva are not known yet, the half-life of Boniva is measured in days and therefore does not stay in your system for years like Fosamax.

Both daily and monthly Boniva users reported the common side effects of bisphosphonates (**Table 10**), but monthly users reported more abdominal pain, joint pain, nausea, and diarrhea than those taking daily Boniva. Intravenous users reported fewer side effects overall.

Table 10   Boniva (ibandronate)

Trade Name (Generic Name) [Manufacturer] How Supplied	Clinical Uses	Contraindications	Most Common Side Effects and Adverse Reactions	Special Considerations
Boniva (ibandronate) [Roche and GlaxoSmithKline] 2.5 mg daily tablets (not widely available) 150 mg monthly tablets 3 mg intravenous solution given every 3 months	Prevention and treatment of postmenopausal osteoporosis	Allergy to bisphosphonates Esophageal abnormalities Low blood calcium Poor kidney function Inability to remain upright for 60 minutes	GI distress (i.e., acid reflux, nausea, vomiting, diarrhea, abdominal pain, flatulence, esophageal ulcer) Bone or muscle pain Get immediate help for difficulty swallowing, midline chest pain, or severe abdominal pain	First bisphosphonate to be available for monthly dosing Take first thing after rising for the day on an empty stomach with a full glass of plain water, remain upright and take no other food or drink for at least 60 minutes 2.5 mg tablets are taken daily; 150 mg tablets are taken once a month; intravenous solution is given 3 mg once every 3 months Use caution if upper gastrointestinal disease (e.g., ulcers or reflux); or kidney disease Do not take calcium, other minerals or milk products within 2 hours of taking Boniva Patient support group called MyBoniva available (call 1-800-4BONIVA) Monthly users report more abdominal pain, joint pain, nausea, and diarrhea than daily users RDA of calcium and vitamin D are also important for increasing BMD, both are needed on the day Boniva is taken (at least 2 hours after Boniva) In very rare cases could increase the risk for osteonecrosis of the jaw following dental surgery

Given the importance of taking these medications exactly as prescribed, a monthly medication is an important option for some people. Boniva's manufacturer has also set up a support group to emphasize the importance of taking the medication once per month. If you are prescribed Boniva, call 1-800-4BONIVA for more information.

You should note that Boniva is different from the other bisphosphonates in that you must be able to sit or stand upright for 60 minutes after taking the oral pill, not just 30 minutes, as required for Actonel and Fosamax. Side effects for Boniva are similar to the other bisphosphonates, with esophageal or intestinal complaints being most common. The risk for stomach upset or ulcer is increased if you take NSAIDs, such as ibuprofen, naproxen, or aspirin, while you are taking Boniva. You should call your clinician if you experience chest pain, difficulty swallowing, or severe midline heartburn.

Betty's comment:

I am 86. Both of my knees have been replaced. When I was diagnosed with osteoporosis, I was unable to take an oral medication. It was suggested to me by my physician specializing in osteoporosis that I might want to get an every-3-month intravenous injection of Boniva.

I don't mind getting the injections every 3 months, as it is much easier on my stomach, and I recently had occasion to find out that the Boniva is working.

After my knees were replaced I was sent to physical therapy. I must be truthful and say that the therapy in the beginning was pure agony and my bottom lip bruised easily from biting it! But now I never think about the steel knees except in an airport.

Since I am now able to exercise on my own, I go to the "gym" three times a week and I work out for a good 45 minutes or more.

My exercises include lifting 3- to 5-pound weights and using the rowing machine for upper body strengthening. I do lunges and exercises to improve my posture and I also ride for a few miles on the stationary bike.

I must admit that I hate walking on the treadmill so I usually bring a book to read. Three weeks ago I started a new novel that was so engrossing, I could not leave it at home. I was happily reading the book when I had to turn a page. Usually when I do this, I take my feet off the moving tread and calmly turn the page. But this time, the book slipped, and I grabbed for it. My foot touched the moving treadmill and I was thrown off onto my right side. I think I uttered a choice expletive, and everyone came running. Slowly they lifted me up. The knees were very painful, and the hip and ankle were not doing well.

Fortunately my orthopedic surgeon is in the same building as the physical therapy gym. He spent a good amount of time x-raying and moving parts of my body. There were no fractures, just a badly bruised hip and ankle and some back pain.

My doctor was very quick to tell me that because I had been exercising so faithfully, I had better tension and muscle tone than he had seen in anyone my age. I have also told my osteoporosis doctor about the fall and we agreed that Boniva was clearly helping my bones.

The wonderful result, after this totally unexpected fall, is that I recovered completely within 10 days. I am headed back to the gym—this time without a book to read on the treadmill!

59. I heard there is a medication given once a year called Reclast (zoledronic acid). Is it like other bisphosphonates?

Reclast (zoledronic acid) is another bisphosphonate available for intravenous (IV) administration. Like Boniva, it is used to treat postmenopausal osteoporosis. Unlike Boniva, IV administration is done only once every 12 months (see **Table 11**). Because it is only given intravenously, Reclast does not include following the complex regimen required for taking oral bisphosphonates. IV administration does require a visit to your clinician's office. To protect your kidneys, you must be well hydrated prior to receiving your yearly dose of Reclast, which means drinking lots of water and sometimes getting extra fluids through the IV before receiving the medication. The 5 mg of Reclast comes in an IV bag of 100 milliliters of fluid (a little over 3 ounces), and administration takes about 15 to 20 minutes.

Reclast is very effective in reducing vertebral fractures. Clinical studies showed that it reduced new vertebral fractures by about 75% when compared to placebo. It also reduced new fractures in the hips and at other sites by 25% to 35%.

Some patients are reluctant to try Reclast because they are concerned about the needle insertion needed for IV administration. Usually the nurses giving Reclast are very skilled in doing IV medication administration and it is over before you know it. For many people, the once-a-year administration schedule overrides any concerns about the need for IV administration because it does not require daily, weekly, monthly, or every-3-months administration that can sometimes be hard to follow or remember.

Table 11 Reclast (zoledronic acid)

Trade Name (Generic Name) [Manufacturer] How Supplied	Clinical Uses	Contraindications	Most Common Side Effects and Adverse Reactions	Special Considerations
Reclast (zoledronic acid) [Novartis Pharmaceuticals Corp.] Intravenous solution	Treatment of postmenopausal osteoporosis	Allergy to bisphosphonates Low blood calcium Poor kidney function Pregnancy, breastfeeding	Low blood calcium levels Bone or muscle pain Headache, flu-like symptoms (fever, muscle pain, etc.) Intestinal upset (stomach upset, diarrhea, constipation)	Intravenous solution is given 5 mg once every 12 months following hydration Use caution if kidney disease, dehydration, low blood volume, using agents toxic to kidneys, impaired mineral metabolism, thyroid/parathyroid surgery, hypoparathyroidism, malabsorption, small intestine removed, cancer, recent chemotherapy, corticosteroid use, poor oral hygiene, asthma, aspirin sensitivity RDA of calcium and vitamin D are also important for increasing BMD; both are needed each day In very rare cases, could increase the risk for osteonecrosis of the jaw following dental surgery

Reclast was well tolerated in a study done with patients who had recently experienced a low-trauma hip fracture. Patients receiving Reclast were less likely to have adverse events or die than those receiving placebo. Patients receiving Reclast also had significantly fewer fractures. A study evaluating more than 7700 postmenopausal women with osteoporosis also showed that the medication was very well tolerated and that fractures were reduced.

Reclast is also FDA-approved for treatment of Paget's disease (see Question 60). Another form of zoledronic acid, known as Zometa, is used in higher doses with more frequent administration for bone cancers, multiple myeloma, and high blood calcium levels associated with some types of cancer. Recent research suggests that Zometa may also be helpful in reducing breast cancer recurrences and metastases. Reclast is not used in combination with other osteoporosis medications.

60. Didronel (etidronate) is usually prescribed for Paget's disease. Is it ever prescribed for osteoporosis?

Didronel (etidronate) is another bisphosphonate. It is FDA-approved for Paget's disease, high calcium levels related to cancer, and rare bone conditions related to hip replacement surgery, but not for osteoporosis. Outside of the United States, Didronel is used for osteoporosis. It works a little differently from other bisphosphonates in that it kills off the osteoclasts (the cells that break down bone). Nonetheless, Didronel has been very effective in reducing osteoporosis-related fractures, particularly spinal ones, and safety has been established for 7 years or more use in postmenopausal women. Additionally, like other bisphosphonates, some protective effects of Didronel on bone density have been shown to persist even after stopping the medication. Didronel is not FDA-approved for treatment or prevention of osteoporosis in the United States.

Paget's disease
Causes large, deformed bones due to the excessive breakdown and formation of bone. Although totally unrelated to osteoporosis, it can occur with osteoporosis in the same bones.

Although **Paget's disease** is also a bone disease, it is totally unrelated to osteoporosis. One person can have both conditions. Paget's disease causes large, deformed bones because of an excessive breakdown and formation of bone. The most common presenting symptom is bone pain located where the bone is closest to a joint. Paget's disease can often be mistaken for arthritis because it is usually diagnosed in people who are over 40 years of age. However, x-rays of bones in individuals with Paget's disease show a characteristic pattern and fractures occur frequently. Blood levels of alkaline phosphatase are usually elevated in people with Paget's disease. If the skull bone is affected, hearing loss can result.

The treatment of choice for Paget's is a bisphosphonate. Bisphosphonates Actonel, Fosamax, Reclast, and Didronel are FDA-approved for the treatment of Paget's. Unlike the longer dosing regimens of other bisphosphonates, Didronel is generally prescribed for only 2 weeks to 3 months at a time depending on the dosage, with a rest period off the medication lasting at least 3 months. This regimen is usually repeated for about 2 years. Didronel is taken on an empty stomach without eating or drinking for 2 hours after taking it. Didronel should still be prescribed with caution in those with upper intestinal disorders. The most common side effects include nausea, diarrhea, and flatulence. Medications that cause stomach upset, such as NSAIDs like ibuprofen, naproxen, or aspirin, can increase the risk for ulcer or heartburn. **Table 12** has information on Didronel.

Table 12 Didronel (etidronate)

Trade Name (Generic Name) [Manufacturer] How Supplied	Clinical Uses	Contraindications	Most Common Side Effects and Adverse Reactions	Special Considerations
Didronel (etidronate) [Procter & Gamble] 200 and 400 mg tablets Also given as an IV injection after hip replacement surgery	Paget's disease Hypercalcemia related to cancer Bone healing problems associated with hip replacement surgery and spinal cord injuries	Allergy or sensitivity to etidronate Severe kidney disease Inability to remain upright for 2 hours Esophageal abnormalities	GI upset (pain, nausea, acid reflux) Bone pain and tenderness Skin rash Other adverse reactions (i.e., seizures, difficulty breathing, and fever have also been reported in IV use)	Although it is a bisphosphonate, it works by causing toxins to destroy some of the bone-breakdown cells (osteoclasts) Taken with plain water on an empty stomach with no food or drink for 2 hours Originally intended for the treatment of Paget's disease After taking Didronel, wait 2 hours before taking calcium and vitamin D Can cause decreased levels of calcium in the blood Prescribed in cycles of daily treatment of 400 mg daily for 2 weeks out of every 3 months for 2 years Not quite as effective as other bisphosphonates for increasing BMD In very rare cases could increase the risk for osteonecrosis of the jaw following dental surgery

Lifestyle Changes and Treatments

147

61. What is Evista® (raloxifene)? What is a SERM, and why is it effective in the treatment of osteoporosis?

Evista (raloxifene) is the only FDA-approved estrogen agonist/antagonist for the prevention and treatment of osteoporosis in postmenopausal women. Evista used to be called a selective estrogen receptor modulator (or SERM), until September 2007 when the FDA changed the name for this class of medications to estrogen agonist/antagonist. Many clinicians still use the term "SERM." You may be more familiar with tamoxifen, an estrogen agonist/antagonist used in the treatment of breast cancer. An estrogen agonist/antagonist binds with some estrogen receptor sites around the body. Although raloxifene is not a hormone, it has an estrogen-like effect in some body tissues such as bone and has an estrogen-blocking effect on other tissues such as breast and uterus.

Evista increases BMD decreases the risk of fractures, and is FDA-approved for the prevention and treatment of osteoporosis in postmenopausal women. The dosage of Evista for both osteoporosis treatment and prevention is 60 mg per day taken as one tablet. Evista, unlike the bisphosphonates, may be taken with or without food. In addition to Evista's positive effects on bone, it also decreases low-density lipoprotein (LDL) cholesterol (the "bad" cholesterol) as well as total cholesterol, but may actually increase triglyceride levels and therefore should be used with caution in women with preexisting high triglycerides and should not be used for prevention of heart disease. Evista reduces the risk for developing breast cancer and is FDA-approved for reducing risk for invasive breast cancer among postmenopausal women with osteoporosis and among postmenopausal women with high risk for invasive breast cancer. Evista's positive effects on bone do not last. Once treatment is stopped, bone loss will resume.

Major side effects seen with Evista are blood clots and stroke. Therefore, the FDA has required a black-box warning on Evista product information identifying these risks. For this reason it is contraindicated in women with a history of blood clots in veins or arteries. Evista can also cause hot flashes. If you already have hot flashes associated with postmenopause, you may want to consider a different medication for osteoporosis. You should not take Evista if you are on either estrogen therapy (ET) or estrogen-progestin therapy (EPT). Evista, however, might be prescribed with a bisphosphonate by a specialist (see Question 67). Evista may represent a good option for post-menopausal women who are not experiencing significant menopausal symptoms or are reluctant to go on ET or EPT for the prevention or treatment of osteoporosis, especially if they have concerns about breast cancer (see Questions 64–66).

If you already have hot flashes associated with postmenopause, you may want to consider a different medication for osteoporosis.

Evista is contraindicated in premenopausal women, women of childbearing age, in pregnancy, and in children, although there is a clinical trial evaluating the effect of Evista on endometriosis in women who are aged 18 to 45. Evista should never be given during pregnancy. Evista is not FDA-approved for use in premenopausal women.

A recent 3-year study of women taking 120 mg of Evista per day showed a 33% decrease in the risk for mild cognitive impairment (mental activities of thinking, learning, and memory). In this study, women taking the usual dosage of 60 mg per day did not see any improvement. The benefits were only found in those taking a double dosage (120 mg) daily. While mild cognitive impairment can be a precursor to Alzheimer's, this study did not show a reduction in cases of Alzheimer's; Alzheimer's takes longer than 3 years to develop. More information about Evista is in **Table 13**.

62. My clinician wants me to give myself injections of something called Forteo® (teriparatide), which I understand to be parathyroid hormone. Should I take it? How often would I receive an injection?

Forteo (teriparatide) is the only currently FDA-approved anabolic agent used in the treatment of osteoporosis. It actually builds bone, in contrast to antiresorptive agents, which interfere with bone resorption by slowing bone breakdown. Forteo builds new bone by increasing the number of osteoblasts (cells that build bone). And it does that in as little as 3 months of daily treatments.

Forteo is a synthetic form of parathyroid hormone, a naturally occurring hormone critical to bone development (see Question 8). Forteo is approved for treating postmenopausal osteoporosis in women who are at high risk for fracture and for increasing bone mass in men with primary (osteoporosis related to aging) or hypogonadal osteoporosis (osteoporosis caused by hypogonadism, which results from inadequate function of the testes and low testosterone levels) who are at high risk for fracture. Forteo is also approved for the treatment of steroid-induced osteoporosis in women and men at high risk for fracture. Those at high risk for fractures include men and women who have a history of osteoporotic fracture, who have multiple risk factors for fracture, for whom other therapies have not worked,

Table 13 Evista (raloxifene)

Trade Name (Generic Name) [Manufacturer] How Supplied	Clinical Uses	Contraindications	Most Common Side Effects and Adverse Reactions	Special Considerations
Evista (raloxifene) [Lilly] 60 mg tablets	Prevention and treatment of postmenopausal osteoporosis Prevention of invasive breast cancer in postmenopausal women with osteoporosis Prevention of invasive breast cancer among postmenopausal women at high risk	Sensitivity to drug or class Taking or using oral or topical systemic therapies containing estrogen History of blood clots Men and premenopausal women, women of childbearing age, children, pregnancy Severe liver disease	Leg cramps Hot flashes Report signs of blood clots immediately: • pain or warmth in the legs • shortness of breath • coughing up blood or severe chest pain • sudden change in vision Infection, flu-like symptoms, inflammation of mouth/throat, cough, sinusitis Joint pain Nausea Weight gain Depression Rash Insomnia Stomach upset	Not an estrogen; not a hormone; classified as an estrogen agonist/antagonist Taken daily Reduces the risk of breast cancer; does not increase the risk of uterine cancer Risk of blood clots and stroke increased Lowers LDL ("bad" cholesterol) levels and total cholesterol levels but should be used with caution in women with a history of high triglyceride levels; not used for prevention of heart disease Risk of mild cognitive impairment (a precursor to Alzheimer's) was reduced when taking 120 mg per day If you are going to be immobile for any length of time, you should stop Evista for as long as you are immobile to prevent blood clots from forming Because of the hot flash side effect, may want to reconsider taking if you already have moderate-to-severe hot flashes associated with postmenopause Should be used with caution in women with liver disease or those taking cholestyramine, a medication used to reduce cholesterol and bile acids from the blood If you are taking warfarin or Coumadin, your clinician may suggest taking tests for clotting prior to taking Evista RDA of calcium and vitamin D are also important for increasing BMD; both are needed on the day Evista is taken (at least 2 hours after Evista)

or who are intolerant of other osteoporosis therapies. Clinical trials showed that Forteo increased bone density in 94% to 96% of patients and decreased the risk of spinal fractures by 65% and other fractures by 53% in women.

But Forteo has some drawbacks. The FDA has required a "black-box warning" on the Forteo labeling to indicate concern that Forteo may cause osteosarcoma, a rare form of bone cancer. Although no humans developed bone cancer during clinical trials, laboratory rats did develop the disease after receiving Forteo in dosages that were 3 to 60 times higher than those used in humans. The manufacturer, Eli Lilly and Company, is funding a 10-year study to determine if Forteo does cause bone cancer in humans. Using Forteo for longer than 2 years is currently not recommended.

Injection

Given into the muscle or fat tissue or vein using a needle with a syringe attached.

Forteo is taken by self-**injection** each day from a pre-filled syringe-type "pen" containing about 1 month's worth of medication. After 28 days, the pen is discarded even if there are remaining doses. Each pen contains only 3 milliliters of fluid (a little over $\frac{1}{2}$ teaspoon) and 750 micrograms of the synthetic parathyroid hormone. Although larger doses can be prescribed, the recommended daily dosage is about 20 micrograms. You must store your pen in the refrigerator. If it becomes cloudy or contains particles, do not use it. The contents of the pen should be clear and colorless. Although some people are squeamish about needles, the needle used in the pen is very, very small.

When you are prescribed Forteo, Lilly and Co. provides you with a starter kit that contains an instructional video.

Occasionally patients develop redness and swelling at the injection site, which is in the fat under the skin of either the thigh or the abdomen. If redness spreads, you should report this to your clinician. The most common side effects are nausea, dizziness, and leg cramps, although other side effects such as low blood pressure, weakness, joint pain, fainting, and chest pain can occur.

Forteo is more expensive than any of the anti-resorptive therapies. But based on your individual case, you may benefit more from Forteo. If you and your clinician decide that you need to take it, be sure to check with your insurance carrier. The manufacturers of Forteo have a customer service center, and they may be able to assist you in getting the medication covered. Without insurance, Forteo can cost about $650 to $850 per month. Lilly has a patient assistance program called Lilly Cares®. Patients who cannot afford their medication can apply for assistance online or by submitting a form via mail. In some instances, patients can get their medications for no charge.

A clinical trial is under way to evaluate Forteo as an effective treatment option in women who have used either Fosamax or Actonel without success. In a study of women who had taken either Fosamax or Evista for almost 3 years, the women who had been on Evista and switched to Forteo built more bone mineral density, and more quickly, than the women who were switched from Fosamax to Forteo. Evista followed by Forteo was more effective than Fosamax followed by Forteo. **Table 14** contains further information about Forteo.

Maggie's comment:

The two prior medications I took for osteoporosis had not helped my bones. In fact, a pair of bone density tests in the

Table 14   Forteo (teriparatide)

Trade Name (Generic Name) [Manufacturer] How Supplied	Clinical Uses	Contraindications	Most Common Side Effects and Adverse Reactions	Special Considerations
Forteo (teriparatide) [Lilly] 20 microgram daily injection from a pen-like syringe containing 3 mL	Treatment of post-menopausal osteoporosis in women at high risk for frac-tures; includes women with a history of osteoporotic fracture, who have multiple risk factors, who have not responded to or are intoler-ant of previous osteoporosis therapy Men with primary osteo-porosis or hypogonadal osteoporosis Treatment of steroid-induced osteoporosis in women and men with high fracture risk.	Paget's disease Unexplained high levels of alkaline phosphatase Children Bone cancer or metastases to the bone Certain bone diseases High blood calcium levels Pregnancy or breastfeeding Allergy to Forteo during previous courses of treatment	Dizziness Leg cramps After each of the first few injections, may experience elevated heart rate or light-headedness; sit or lie down if this happens; report con-tinued symptoms to your clinician Watch for signs of hypercal-cemia: constipation, low energy, nausea, vomiting, or muscle weakness Although no instances of bone cancer have occurred in humans, bone cancer has occurred in rats treated with very high doses	Should not be prescribed for the prevention of osteoporosis Usually reserved for use in people who have not responded to or cannot tolerate other treatments for osteoporosis Decreases risk of fracture in women Fracture risk not yet studied in men Pen must be refrigerated but not frozen, and protected from the light Recap the pen after every use Discard safely after 28 days Rotate sites of injection Safety of using Forteo for longer than 2 years is not known Currently being evaluated in long-term study to determine whether Forteo is linked to a rare form of bone cancer in humans (to date, only occurs in rats that are given 3 to 60 times the human dose) RDA of calcium and vitamin D are also important for increasing BMD; Forteo can raise calcium levels in the blood, so calcium blood levels are sometimes monitored

same month gave nearly identical results: I am 60 but I had the bones of an 85-year-old!

I was referred to an endocrinologist who ordered blood tests to check my vitamin D levels, which were fine. The recommendation: Forteo, an injectable medication that speeds up the renewal of bone. According to the insert with the Forteo syringe, there are two sets of cells in bone: set #1 breaks down old bone, and set #2 builds it back up again. Ideally, these two sets work in synch; in my case, the second set was "slacking"!

There is a recommended treatment span of 2 years. As there is a black-box warning of bone cancer with this medication, I am looking for any sign of improvement after the first year of treatment, which will (hopefully) be confirmed with a bone density test. The doctor feels that Forteo will certainly prevent further deterioration and, "if we hit a home run," the damage may be reversed. Meanwhile, I inject myself daily and look forward to hearing better news this year than last.

63. I have a very small fracture in one of the bones in my back. I've been prescribed Miacalcin® (calcitonin) in a nasal spray. What is Miacalcin? Can a nasal spray be effective for treating a bone fracture? Is Fortical® (calcitonin) nasal spray the same as Miacalcin?

Calcitonin is a hormone secreted by the nonthyroid cells in the thyroid gland that plays an important role in maintaining bone strength and regulating blood levels of calcium. Manufactured calcitonin is sold under the trade names of Miacalcin and Fortical. Miacalcin Nasal Spray and Fortical (calcitonin-salmon) are manufactured forms of calcitonin with action essentially identical to those made in the body but with greater potency and longer duration. They have the same amino acids as the calcitonin found in salmon, which is why they're often designated as calcitonin-salmon. Calcitonin is one of the earliest discovered treatments for osteoporosis. Formerly given as a subcutaneous injection, Miacalcin NS is now taken as a once-a-day nasal spray. Fortical is also a once-a-day nasal spray, but has never been available as a subcutaneous injection. Calcitonin decreases osteoclasts to prevent further bone breakdown.

Miacalcin NS and Fortical are indicated in the treatment of low bone mass in women who have been in postmenopause for at least 5 years or for whom estrogen is not an option. The PROOF (Prevent Recurrence of Osteoporotic Fractures) Trial showed that 200 IU per day of Miacalcin reduced spinal fractures by 33%; however, 5 years of treatment with Miacalcin did not reduce overall fracture rates. Surprisingly, even women who took 400 IU of Miacalcin did not have reduced fracture risk, but because many women did not complete the study, the results may have been distorted. According to Miacalcin's prescribing information, it does not increase BMD in other bones besides the spine. Studies evaluating Fortical similarly demonstrated increases in bone density at the spine.

Calcitonin has been used successfully for pain relief in women who have had spinal fractures, although it is not FDA-approved as an analgesic. While few studies have evaluated pain relief with calcitonin, many personal reports of pain relief support this use. It is often taken at bedtime because calcitonin nasal spray gets into your system rapidly and reaches peak blood levels in 30 minutes. When taken as a nasal spray, it is used as one spray in one nostril every day, alternating nostrils daily. The nasal spray is dispensed from a pump and bottle. The pump must be primed before using for the first time, but it should not be primed before each dose. Unopened bottles should be stored in a refrigerator but not frozen. Before the first dose of the 30-dose container is used, the contents should reach room temperature, and the remaining amount should then be stored at room temperature.

So, although Miacalcin and Fortical (calcitonin) can be prescribed for postmenopausal osteoporosis, they are rarely the first choice for osteoporosis-related fractures. Instead, calcitonin is usually used in combination with other therapies (such as estrogen or estrogen agonists/antagonists), and most often following a vertebral fracture for its pain-relieving effects. Like all prescription therapies for osteoporosis prevention and treatment, calcitonin nasal spray should be taken with calcium and adequate vitamin D. Consideration for medication cost must also be weighed, as long-term therapy with Miacalcin NS can cost thousands of dollars per year. See a summary of Miacalcin NS's and Fortical's indications, side effects, and special considerations in **Table 15**.

Penny's comment:

When you stop to think about it, cleaning up after dinner is not usually a difficult task. But as I leaned into the refrigerator, I felt the pain in my back. I couldn't breathe or scream. Bent over and twisted sideways, I finally made it to my bed. By then I could scream for the heating pad and two Aleve tablets.

The next morning, I was off to see my orthopedic doctor (every person over 65 should have one), who told me that

Table 15 Miacalcin Nasal Spray and Fortical (calcitonin-salmon)

Trade Name (Generic Name) [Manufacturer] How Supplied	Clinical Uses	Contraindications	Most Common Side Effects and Adverse Reactions	Special Considerations
Miacalcin NS (calcitonin-salmon) [Novartis] Nasal spray 3.7 milliliter/bottle; each dose contains about 200 IU of calcitonin	Postmenopausal women who have osteoporosis (in postmenopause >5 years)	Allergy to calcitonin-salmon	Nasal stuffiness Dry mouth Nausea Nosebleeds Headache	Interferes with osteoclasts to reduce bone breakdown Increases BMD in lumbar vertebrae, but not as much as other prescription options for treatment of bone loss
Fortical (calcitonin-salmon) [Unigene] 3.7 milliliter/bottle; each dose contains about 200 IU of calcitonin	Postmenopausal women who have a vertebral (spinal) fracture			Give one spray in one nostril every day; alternate the nostrils Probably provides pain relief in women with vertebral (spinal) fractures; may be more helpful in this regard if given at bedtime Use with caution in women with poor kidney function or pernicious (vitamin B_{12}) anemia Calcitonin sometimes given as injection for Paget's disease of bone

I had a compression fracture of the thoracic vertebra #5. Getting on and lying on the x-ray table was excruciating.

I was fitted for a brace, made in two sections of stainless steel, one just above the groin area, and the upper steel brace just hitting the top of the breast bone, all connected with a plastic 6-inch-wide belt, suspended between the two steel braces and intended to torture me by keeping my back straight. I looked in the mirror. I bulged in all the wrong places. I looked like an ink blot test waiting to be analyzed— bumps and ridges never before a part of my torso.

I had to wear the brace during the day for about 6 weeks. My doctor prescribed Miacalcin nasal spray and some pain medication. Although I later learned that this fracture indicated that I have osteoporosis, I wasn't told that at the time. Now I need to be more aware of what I can and cannot do. I need to learn to bend at the knees, keeping my back straight—no more bending over to put stuff in the refrigerator or the oven! Although I was told that only the first vertebra fracture causes pain, I have since heard that is not true. I just can't believe that a fracture in my spine wouldn't hurt every time it happens!

64. I've reached menopause and my clinician wants to treat my hot flashes with estrogen because estrogen will also help prevent more bone loss. Is this true?

Estrogen therapy (ET) is the single most effective treatment for moderate vasomotor symptoms associated with menopause. **Vasomotor symptoms**, which include hot flashes and night sweats, are a direct result of low levels of estrogen that occur during perimenopause and postmenopause (see Question 9).

Vasomotor symptoms

Symptoms resulting from irregular functioning of the part of the brain that controls body heat, usually experienced as hot flashes and sweats that may or may not be followed by feeling cold or chilled.

Vasomotor symptoms can start during perimenopause, the time period leading up to menopause, including the 12 months of no menses, when symptoms of hormonal changes occur. But if you only have an occasional hot flash or if you don't find daily hot flashes bothersome, then your symptoms probably don't require estrogen for treatment. If your symptoms are moderate to severe, then estrogen therapy might be a good option for both vasomotor symptom relief and bone protection. If you have a uterus, then you would need to take estrogen plus progestin therapy (EPT). The progestin protects the lining of the uterus from overgrowth, which can lead to endometrial cancer.

Estrogen is very effective in preventing and treating bone loss. Once you reach menopause, your bone loss becomes very rapid. You may lose as much as 5% of your bone density every year in the 4 to 8 years following menopause. Estrogen was FDA-approved for the management of osteoporosis back in 1972. More recently, the indication was changed to prevention of osteoporosis; however, it is not FDA-approved for treatment of osteoporosis. Studies of postmenopausal women taking estrogen for 1 year indicate that their bone density increases in their hip, spine, and forearm. Findings also indicate that the type of estrogen does not matter. All types of estrogen, including **conjugated equine estrogen**, **bioidentical** estradiol, or synthetic estrogens, provide bone protection and help to increase bone mineral density.

While there was good evidence that bone density increased, it was not so clear whether estrogen actually reduced fracture rates until the Women's Health Initiative (WHI). The WHI was a very large study of thousands of postmenopausal women whose average

Conjugated equine estrogen

The most common form of estrogen used in hormone therapy (HT), extracted from the urine of pregnant mares.

Bioidentical

Refers to hormones manufactured in a laboratory, usually from wild yam or soy, that have the exact same chemical makeup as the hormones made in the body; also termed "natural" hormones.

age was about 63. The original intent of the study, which was started in 1991, was to research the cardio-vascular effects of estrogen therapy or estrogen prog-estin therapy on postmenopausal women.

The clinicians and the women in the WHI were "blinded" in that they did not know whether a study participant was taking estrogen or a placebo. Older postmenopausal women without significant vasomotor symptoms were chosen because women in post-menopause who had hot flashes or night sweats would know that they were taking a drug instead of a placebo if the flashes or sweats went away.

The study results were also used to show the effect of estrogen on osteoporotic fractures. There was very good news for women's bones: Researchers found that fracture risk was reduced in both of the estrogen groups (also called "arms" of the study). In fact, spine and hip fractures were reduced by 33%. Although estrogen clearly demon-strated its positive effect on bone during the WHI, the estrogen progestin therapy arm of the study was stopped 3 years earlier than planned because of increased risk of breast cancer, heart disease, dementia, stroke, and clots. The estrogen-only arm was also stopped about 1 year early, not because it increased the risk of breast cancer but because estrogen alone also increased a woman's risk of stroke and clots (see Question 66).

The FDA now requires black-box warnings on all estrogen products for these effects, plus the risk of endometrial cancer. Endometrial cancer can be pre-vented with the use of progesterone in women who have their uterus (see Question 66). Also according to the black-box warning, menopause hormone therapy (MHT) is not to be used for preventing heart disease or dementia.

Don't forget that the WHI study participants were generally older. When the data were reanalyzed by looking at women in various age groups, the risks for heart disease were not increased in women immediately following menopause. The WHI data reanalysis supported findings from prior meta-analyses that showed using MHT immediately after menopause did not increase risks for heart disease (see Question 66).

So, yes, taking estrogen will not only help to prevent bone loss, it will also increase BMD and decrease your risk of fractures. Deciding whether to take MHT which customarily refers to either ET or EPT, is a very important decision for your overall health. If you do not have moderate-to-severe vasomotor symptoms, you should not take MHT solely to prevent osteoporosis. But if you need relief from your symptoms, you and your clinician should decide if the benefits of MHT outweigh the risks of taking it for you.

Faith's comment:

I started menopause in my 40s—first the hot flashes and erratic periods, followed by mood swings. Because of my age and the fact that I had been on a medication for hypertension for a number of years, my gynecologist believed that menopause hormone therapy (MHT) was necessary to lessen the risk of heart disease and to keep my bones strong, since my mother has osteoporosis and I am small-boned. Although I was reluctant to begin MHT, the hot flashes, sleep deprivation, and incredible mood swings had worn me down. I wanted to be me again—fairly easy-going— not this person I no longer recognized. I took the MHT and experienced great relief. My bone test showed strong bones. All was great until the Women's Health Initiative study was released! Frightened, I stopped MHT.

Within 6 months my bone scan revealed osteopenia—worse in my spine, less severe in my hips. My gynecologist encouraged me to increase my calcium supplements, do weight-bearing exercises, and walk. I walked, lost weight, increased my calcium supplements to 1600 mg/day, and did free weights. I felt great. My bone scan the following year showed a slight improvement in my hips, but a worsening of my spine. Interestingly, I had also noticed that my posture seemed to be worsening . . . and that I seemed to constantly remind myself to stand up straight.

Looking back, I think my diet as a teenager and preadolescent was horrible—not much calcium (unless you count ice cream!) and meals that consisted of fries and Coke. I don't think I gave my bones much of a fighting chance.

My gynecologist recommended Fosamax, but I wanted a chance to try to improve my spine. However, a few months later when I had a physical by my nurse practitioner, she was adamant that I begin Fosamax immediately. She felt that my spine showed osteoporosis and that I was at risk of fractures. I began Fosamax. I'm curious to see what my next bone test looks like.

65. What about the new low-dose hormone patch, Menostar® (estradiol), that is used to prevent osteoporosis?

Menostar (estradiol) was FDA-approved in 2004 for the prevention of postmenopausal osteoporosis. It is a dime-sized transdermal patch that delivers about 14 micrograms of estrogen per day. A new patch is applied every week. Because your body absorbs the estrogen from the patch through the skin, you can avoid the liver "first-pass" effect, meaning that the hormone is not metabolized through your liver. Instead, it can go directly into the bloodstream.

The estrogen that is used in this patch is estradiol, one of the three estrogens made by the human body. Estradiol is the one in greatest abundance until menopause. Then levels drop off to near zero. Although estrone, another of the three estrogens, continues to be circulated in both men and women, it is not sufficient in quantity to prevent bone loss. Estradiol in Menostar is derived from plants but is bioidentical to the estradiol in the human body, meaning it is the exact, or identical, chemical structure as the estradiol made by your body. While manufactured estradiol is a bioidentical hormone, it still carries with it the same risks and benefits of other manufactured estrogens that have been studied more completely, such as conjugated equine estrogens. (See Questions 64 and 66 for further discussion of the risks and benefits of taking estrogen.)

The blood levels of estrogen resulting from Menostar are high enough to preserve bone. Research shows that Menostar is also effective for treating vasomotor symptoms associated with menopause. Menostar is not FDA-approved for vasomotor symptom treatment, and since it is such a low dose, some women may need higher estrogen doses to manage their individual symptoms. The blood levels of estrogen generated by hormone therapy that is usually used to treat vasomotor symptoms are two to eight times higher than those generated by Menostar.

If you are postmenopausal and want to prevent osteoporosis, or if you have osteopenia and you want to prevent further bone loss, Menostar may be appropriate for you. Menostar is not FDA-approved for osteoporosis treatment. Other treatment options are used instead.

Like all estrogen preparations that are of sufficient strength to raise blood levels, contraindications to Menostar include breast cancer or any estrogen-dependent cancer, history of stroke or heart attack (myocardial infarction), abnormal uterine bleeding, and a history of or current blood clot(s). **Table 16** summarizes Menostar.

66. There is a lot of controversy about taking estrogen. Why is that? Should I accept the risks of being on it so that I can prevent further bone loss?

When the WHI estrogen-progestin (the participants were taking PremPro) arm of the study was halted in 2002, media concentrated on what causedresearchers to stop the study prematurely. The researchers found that the risk of breast cancer, stroke, cardiovascular events, and clots outweighed the benefits of fewer colorectal cancers and fewer hip fractures. In 2004, the estrogen-only arm of the study was also stopped prematurely, but not because of the risk of breast cancer. The researchers determined that the risk of stroke and clots was high enough to warrant stopping the study 1 year earlier than planned.

The increased risk of getting breast cancer while taking daily EPT (0.625 mg of conjugated equine estrogens and 2.5 mg of medroxyprogesterone) was reported as 26%. But that kind of statistic is more alarming than helpful. Using the WHI study's design and results, one could predict that of 10,000 postmenopausal women who were taking a placebo, 30 of them would develop breast cancer. If you looked at 10,000 postmenopausal women who were taking EPT

Table 16 Menostar (estradiol)

Trade Name (Generic Name) [Manufacturer] How Supplied	Clinical Uses	Contraindications	Most Common Side Effects and Adverse Reactions	Special Considerations
Menostar (estradiol) [Berlex] Transdermal patch (delivers 14 micrograms per day)	Osteoporosis prevention in postmenopausal women	Men Breast cancer Estrogen-dependent cancer History of blood clots Current blood vessel inflammation or blood clot History of stroke or heart attack Abnormal undiagnosed uterine bleeding	Patch site irritation Joint pain Vaginal discharge/ bleeding Breast changes Nausea/vomiting Headaches Rash Hair changes	The estrogen used in this patch is plant-derived estradiol, which is bioidentical to one of the estrogens made naturally in your body Has half of the estrogen used in most other transdermal patches—is successful in the prevention of osteoporosis and may prevent vasomotor symptoms Significantly increases bone mineral density after 2 years Length of treatment should be weighed carefully with risks associated with all estrogens Apply new patch weekly Apply to clean and dry skin, usually the upper arm or on the abdomen; do not apply on or near breast Not necessary to take progestin regularly, but you should discuss with your clinician the need for taking progestin two times per year for 14 days to allow uterine lining to shed (like a menstrual period); women without a uterus do not need to take progestin The dosage of estrogen in Menostar is not enough to prevent hot flashes and night sweats

Also see Table 17; all estrogens carry the same contraindications, side effects, and potential reactions.

for 5 or more years, 38 of them would develop breast cancer. The difference between 30 and 38 represents a 26% increase, but still only 8 more women out of 10,000 would develop breast cancer. If you happen to become 1 of the 8 (or 38 total), it's an important statistic to consider when making a decision. However, the media tended to jump on the increased risk of breast cancer; many women, when hearing this news, stopped their hormones cold-turkey. Many clinicians stopped prescribing hormones entirely.

After much more analysis of the WHI data as it applied to the EPT arm, there was more discussion among researchers and clinicians. Three points of view tended to develop from further analysis and discussion. One viewpoint was that the study was faulty in its design and conclusions, so we should not pay attention to the results. For example, the women who took part in the WHI study were well into their postmenopausal years and did not have significant vasomotor symptoms. Questions arise from this observation. Do women earlier in postmenopause develop the same risks? Because breast cancer takes as long as 7 years to develop, another question arises: Is it fair to attribute increased breast cancer risk to taking EPT for only 5 years? The second viewpoint was more absolute. No one should go on hormones, or hormones would have to be the last resort for treatment of menopausal symptoms. The third viewpoint falls somewhere in the middle, that the WHI brought important information to light about hormones but that there is still a place for the use of hormones in the treatment of the moderate-to-severe symptoms of menopause.

The controversy has not stopped. The estrogen-alone arm of the WHI showed a small decrease in the risk of breast cancer, which raised questions about the role of progestins in the development of breast cancer. More recently, there was an analysis of many studies in which women used ET or EPT. The result of looking at all of those data showed that estrogen is still an important treatment option for moderate-to-severe menopausal symptoms, and that the risk of death from heart disease or cancer was not increased when MHT is started in the early postmenopausal years. The WHI data were reanalyzed to look at effects for women in various age groups and found similar results. Younger women, who had just passed through menopause, did not have the increased risks for heart disease that were seen among older women. These results have shifted thinking again, and many more clinicians are now prescribing MHT for women immediately after menopause. MHT, like any medication, should be used in the lowest dose and for the shortest period of time possible.

The decision to use MHT can be a difficult one. With regard to your bones, you should not take it for the treatment of bone loss unless you have moderate-to-severe hot flashes or night sweats that require treatment. The smallest dose that will help your symptoms should be used. Any estrogen used orally or transdermally (by cream, gel, spray, mousse, or patch) will improve your bone density. Using vaginal estrogen for vaginal dryness will probably not provide you with enough estrogen to protect your bones, unless you use a vaginal estrogen ring such as Femring (estradiol). The Menostar patch protects your bones and may also treat your vasomotor symptoms.

Although MHT can prevent postmenopausal osteoporosis and is often used together with bisphosphonates or calcitonin, it is not an approved treatment for established osteoporosis. You should use other non-estrogen medications if you already have osteoporosis. When the long-term effects of estrogen therapy were compared with those of Fosamax (alendronate), improved BMD persisted longer in women taking Fosamax. Table 16 (Question 65) describes Menostar and **Table 17** summarizes other estrogen therapies.

Before taking MHT, you should consider the possible benefits such as menopausal symptom management (including vasomotor symptoms, vaginal dryness, sleep and mood disturbances), osteoporosis prevention, and reduced risks for colon cancer as well as potential risks, including breast cancer, heart disease or stroke, and blood clots. Here are some questions to consider:

- What is the severity of my symptoms? How frequently do they occur? Do they interfere with my work or enjoyment of the activities of daily living?
- Have I kept track of things that bring on symptoms and tried to eliminate them (e.g., stopped eating chocolate if it brings on a hot flash)?
- Am I willing to make changes in my lifestyle to reduce my symptoms?
- What changes have I made in my lifestyle to reduce my symptoms?
- Am I trying to live in healthier ways (e.g., quit smoking)?
- What am I not willing or able to do at this time to modify my life? What is available to help for the short term and the long term?
- In addition to lifestyle changes, have I tried using vitamins and mineral supplements to help with my symptoms?

Table 17   Estrogen Therapies: Part 1, General Information; Part 2, Specific Products

Part 1:   Clinical Uses, Contraindications, and Common Side Effects of All Estrogen Therapies Listed in Part 2

Clinical uses

- Postmenopausal women who have moderate to severe vasomotor symptoms and/or vaginal atrophy or vaginal dryness
- Prevention of osteoporosis in postmenopausal women with low bone mass or normal bone density who also have other osteoporosis risks and moderate-to-severe vasomotor symptoms
- Postmenopausal women with osteoporosis, but only if they also have moderate-to-severe vasomotor symptoms

Contraindications

- Allergy to estrogen or progesterone or components of tablets, capsules, etc.
- Bi-Est and Tri-Est are contraindicated if you have a peanut allergy
- Abnormal, undiagnosed uterine bleeding
- Estrogen-linked cancers; breast cancer; uterine cancer
- History of blood clots in veins or history of blood clots in arteries within past 12 months
- Pregnancy
- Liver problems

Serious adverse reactions (though rare) include: depression; uterine fibroid growth; worsening of asthma; blood clots; stroke; heart attack; dementia; cancers of the breast, ovary, or uterine lining; problems with gallbladder, liver, or pancreas.

More common reactions include: vaginal bleeding or spotting; slight breast enlargement or thickening; breast soreness; bloating or cramps; weight changes; nausea; vomiting; headache; swelling; high blood pressure; hair thinning or increased hair growth; rash; vaginal yeast infections; vision changes; difficulty wearing contact lenses.

Part 2: Specific Products

Name	Product Contents	Manufacturer	Form(s) Available	Comments
Activella	Estradiol and norethindrone acetate	Novo Nordisk	Tablets	• Combination of progestin and bioidentical estradiol taken daily
Alora	Estradiol	Watson	Transdermal patch	• Biodentical estradiol • Patch may be cut smaller for smaller dosage • Patch is changed twice a week • Do not apply patch to breast
Angeliq	Estradiol and norethindrone	Bayer HealthCare Pharmaceuticals	Tablet	• Estrogen–progestogen combination taken daily
Bi-Est and **Tri-Est**	Estriol and estradiol and Estriol, estradiol, estrone	Various manufacturers at compounding pharmacies	Capsules	• Bi-Est and Tri-Est contain bioidentical hormones manufactured by extracting steroid molecules from soy and wild yam, an herb • Different combinations of the estrogens can be compounded • Tell compounding pharmacy if you have a peanut allergy; peanut oil is used in the capsules
Bi-Est with progesterone* **Tri-Est with progesterone**	Estradiol, estriol, and micronized progesterone Estradiol, estriol, estrone, and micronized progesterone	Compounding pharmacies	Capsules	• Bioidentical hormones • Can be compounded in various strengths and percentages • Tell compounding pharmacy if you have peanut allergy

(*cont.*)

Table 17 Estrogen Therapies: Part 1, General Information; Part 2, Specific Products (*cont.*)

Part 2: Specific Products (*cont.*)

Name	Product Contents	Manufacturer	Form(s) Available	Comments
Cenestin	Synthetic conjugated estrogen	Teva Pharmaceuticals	Tablets	• Plant-derived estrogens
Climara	Estradiol	Bayer HealthCare Pharmaceuticals	Transdermal patch	• Bioidentical estradiol • Patch may be cut smaller to make smaller dosage • Patch changed once a week • Do not apply patch to breast
Climara Pro	Estradiol plus levonorgestral	Bayer HealthCare Parmaceuticals	Transdermal patch	• Patch applied once weekly • Apply to clean, dry skin of lower abdomen; do not apply patch to breast • Rotate sites, avoid waistline • Bioidentical estradiol and synthetic progestin
CombiPatch	Estradiol and norethindrone	Novartis Pharmaceuticals	Transdermal patch	• Both hormones in one patch • Bioidentical estradiol and progestin is synthetic • Comes in two strengths/sizes of patch • Change patches every 3 to 4 days • Use on dry, clean skin; do not apply patch to breast
Depo-Estradiol	Estradiol cypionate	Pfizer	Injection	• Given every 3 to 4 weeks • FDA-approved treatment for hot flashes

Divigel	Estradiol	Upsher-Smith Laboratories	Topical Gel	• Apply one packet daily • Apply to upper thigh • Apply to clean, dry skin
Elestrin	Estradiol	PharmaDerm	Topical Gel	• Apply one pump of gel daily • Apply to upper arm • Apply to clean, dry skin
Enjuvia	Conjugated estrogens, B	Teva Pharmaceuticals	Tablets	• Plant-derived estrogens • Controlled release to provide sustained relief of vasomotor symptoms over a 24-hour period
Estrace	Micronized estradiol	Warner Chilcott	Tablets	• Sometimes placed under the tongue
Estraderm	Estradiol	Novartis	Transdermal patch	• Bioidentical estradiol • Change patch twice a week • Do not cut this patch • Do not apply patch to breast

(cont.)

Table 17 Estrogen Therapies: Part 1, General Information; Part 2, Specific Products (cont.)

Part 2: Specific Products (cont.)

Name	Product Contents	Manufacturer	Form(s) Available	Comments
			Tablets	• Take with food to reduce stomach upset
Estratest HS **Estratest** **(various generics)**	All are esterified estrogens and methytestosterone	Solvay Solvay Varied	Tablets	• Tablet contains both estrogen and testosterone • FDA-approved for treatment of hot flashes when other hormone treatments have not provided relief • Although not FDA-approved for improving libido, this combination often used "off-label" to help both hot flashes and low libido
EstroGel	Estradiol	Ascend Therapeutics, Inc.	Transdermal gel	• Bioidentical estradiol • Gel applied once daily to arm, from shoulder to wrists, like a skin cream • Takes several minutes to dry • Odorless • Measured doses from a non-aerosol pump
Estrasorb	Emulsified estradiol	Esprit Pharma	Cream	• Bioidentical estradiol • Cream rubbed into each thigh with each dose • Takes several minutes to dry • Supplied in packets • Be sure it is fully dry prior to dressing
Evamist	Estradiol	Ther-Rx Corp	Solution	• Apply one spray daily • Apply spray to forearm • Apply to clean, dry skin

FemHRT	Ethinyl estradiol and norenthindrone acetate	Warner Chilcott	Tablets	• Tablet contains estrogen and progesterone taken daily
Femring	Estradiol acetate	Warner Chilcott	Vaginal ring	• If you can feel it inside, it is not positioned correctly • Replaced once every 3 months • Provides enough estrogen to relieve vasomotor symptoms and vaginal dryness • May provide support for urinary incontinence
Femtrace	Estradiol acetate	Warner Chilcott	Tablets	• Taken daily • Take with food as needed to reduce stomach upset
Menest	Esterified estrogen	King Pharmaceutics, Inc.	Tablets	• Also used in the palliative treatment of breast cancer
Menostar	Estradiol	Bayer HealthCare Pharmaceuticals	Patch	• Change patch weekly • Apply to lower abdominal area • FDA-approved for osteoporosis prevention; research shows also effective for vasomotor symptoms associated with menopause
Ogen	Estropipate	Pfizer	Tablets	• Recommended for cyclic regimens 21 days on, 7 days off
Prefest	Estradiol and norgestimate	Teva Pharmaceuticals	Tablets	• Bioidentical estradiol made from soy • Taken daily in sequence: 3 tablets of estradiol, then 3 tablets of estradiol and norgestimate, then repeat

(cont.)

Table 17   Estrogen Therapies: Part 1, General Information; Part 2, Specific Products (*cont.*)

Part 2:   Specific Products (*cont.*)

Name	Product Contents	Manufacturer	Form(s) Available	Comments
Premarin	Conjugated equine estrogen	Wyeth	Tablets	• The most studied estrogen, conjugated equine estrogen CEE is manufactured using estrogens found in pregnant mare's urine
Premphase	Conjugated equine estrogen in 14 tablets, then conjugated equine estrogen plus medroxy-progesterone acetate in 14 tablets	Wyeth	Tablets	• You will get a period when you finish the tablets containing estrogen and progestin • Contains CEE, the most studied estrogen
Prempro	Conjugated equine estrogen and medroxyprogesterone acetate	Wyeth	Tablets	• Available in many dosages • Contains CEE • One tablet containing both estrogen and progestin taken daily
Vivelle-Dot	Estradiol	Novartis	Transdermal patch	• Smallest available patch size to treat menopausal symptoms • Changed twice a week • Do not apply patch to breast

*If you still have a uterus and are taking oral estrogen or some estrogens applied to the skin or vagina, a progestin is needed to protect your uterus lining from overgrowth.

- Do I have any medical conditions that would make it unsafe for me to go on MHT? Am I taking any medications that would interact badly with MHT?
- If I go on hormones, what would be the best route of administration for me? Will I be able to develop a regimen of remembering to take pills? Will I be willing to change patches? Will I be willing to apply vaginal cream or insert a vaginal ring?
- Will I be comfortable knowing that there are risks to taking estrogen and progesterone? Do I understand that all medications, vitamins, herbs, and supplements carry certain risks?
- Do I understand the benefits of estrogen in addition to relieving menopausal symptoms, such as reducing the risk of bone loss and colon cancer?
- Do I understand the side effects of hormone therapy? Do I understand that the hormones may relieve one symptom but that I may get another symptom as a result of the hormones?
- If I took hormones and I stopped having severe hot flashes, how happy would I be? If hormones could relieve the symptoms, do I think my life would be much better?
- Do I understand that taking hormones does not mean that I will get breast cancer? And do I also understand that avoiding hormones does not prevent me from getting breast cancer?

Once you have decided to use MHT for your vasomotor symptoms and your bone health, you should make sure the following questions are answered before you leave with your prescription:

- How long will I be on this drug?
- What symptoms should I report to my clinician?

- When does my clinician want to see me again?
- What are the options if I choose not to take this drug?
- How long will it be before I notice any improvement or change?
- What side effects or symptoms should I watch for? How can I minimize or prevent these symptoms?
- Will side effects or symptoms decrease with time?
- If I don't like taking it, should I let my clinician know I have stopped it?
- What do I do if I miss a dose?
- What if I go out of town and leave my prescription at home? Will it be a problem if I miss a week? A month?
- Is there a specific time of day I should take my medications?
- Will MHT interact with other medications that I'm taking?
- Are there other nonprescription medicines, herbs, or dietary supplements that I should not take with MHT?
- Can I still drink alcohol?

67. Can I take prescription osteoporosis medications in combination with each other? Which medications could I use together to get more improvement in my bones?

In the case of treating osteoporosis, a combination of agents can mean more BMD than is gained by using one agent alone. Because there are no data yet on the risk of fractures, it's not clear if increasing BMD using combination therapies necessarily decreases fracture risk more, which is the goal of combining therapies. Treatment with two drugs is clearly more expensive than treating with one drug alone, and the risk for developing side effects increases. According to the 2004 *Surgeon General's Report on Bone Health*, combination therapies should be reserved for individuals whose bone mass is very low and has not improved on one medication, for those who have a fracture while on one medication, or for those who have very low BMD and a history of multiple fractures. Further, osteoporosis medication should only be taken in combination on the recommendation of a clinician who specializes in the treatment of osteoporosis.

Although bisphosphonates, estrogen agonists/antagonists, and estrogens all prevent bone breakdown, they do this by different actions. This means that some of them can be taken together. And when taken together, the increase in bone density is greater than if the agents are taken alone. However, some combinations oversuppress bone turnover, increasing the risk for developing "**frozen bone**," which means that even though bone mass may increase, the quality of the bone is not good enough to reduce the risk of fractures. Frozen bone may happen when the bone actually becomes more brittle rather than stronger as a result of the action of the medications. For example, taking a combination of Fosamax and Evista or a bisphosphonate and estrogen can increase bone mineral density more than each drug taken separately, but the risk of developing frozen bone due to **oversuppression** of bone turnover is also present. Since few data are available regarding the effects on fracture with combination therapies, combinations are reserved for certain individuals, as previously noted. Fosamax and estrogen were taken together by a group of postmenopausal women with a **hysterectomy**, while two

Frozen bone

Speculated to be a potential concern in individuals taking combinations of osteoporosis medications. While the medications increase bone mass, the bone quality may not be as good, resulting in bone that is more brittle rather than stronger.

Oversuppression

Occurs when bone turnover is suppressed to such a high extent that bone quality may be compromised; associated with "frozen bone."

Hysterectomy

Removal of the uterus.

other groups took one or the other of the two medications. Bone density in the spine and hip increased more in the group taking the combination of therapies than in the groups taking either Fosamax or estrogen alone. However, there was concern that the combination may suppress bone turnover to the point where frozen bone could occur. Similarly, Actonel and MHT also increase bone density when taken individually and taking them together improves bone density even more—however, the quality of the bone remains of concern.

Before deciding with your clinician on a combination approach to preventing and treating osteoporosis, medications should be examined for additional benefits they could provide besides those for your bones. For example, MHT has the benefit of treating the most bothersome symptoms of menopause such as hot flashes, night sweats, and vaginal atrophy. Evista can reduce your risk of breast cancer and heart disease. When taken in combination with bisphosphonates, Evista does not lose these other benefits. However, don't forget that taking two medications means coping with two sets of side effects, the cost of both medications, and potentially negative effects on bone quality.

There are some firm restrictions to using other medications together. Calcitonin nasal spray and bisphosphonates should not be taken together because they may actually oppose one another in their actions. Despite this caution, calcitonin nasal spray is sometimes prescribed following a vertebral fracture for its pain-relieving effects even in those taking bisphosphonates. Forteo (teriparatide) builds bone density when taken by itself, but when taken in combination with Fosamax, bone density does not increase as much as when either agent is taken alone. However, when Fosamax is taken after treatment with Forteo is finished, the improvement in bone density is even greater. So, while taking Fosamax and Forteo together is not helpful, taking Fosamax following treatment with Forteo may provide additional benefit. Again, Evista (raloxifene) and MHT or any estrogen therapies cannot be taken together.

Remember that combination therapy is reserved for individuals whose bone mass is very low and has not improved on one medication, for those who have a fracture while on one medication, or for those who have very low BMD and a history of multiple fractures—and then only on the recommendation of a specialist. The American Association of Clinical Endocrinologists (AACE) advises against using medications in combination with one another until the results of using combinations are analyzed for their effect on fracture risk. The National Osteoporosis Foundation (NOF) recommends caution and carefully considering potential benefits when combining therapies due to the unknown effects of combining medications on fracture risk, increased cost when using two medications, and potential increase in side effects.

68. Are there any medications that are available without a prescription to treat osteoporosis?

Vitamins, minerals, and dietary supplements can be sold over the counter (OTC)—that is, without a prescription. These products can be purchased in drug stores, health food stores, some department stores, and over the Internet. The FDA does not regulate OTC products as they do prescription medications. Because of this, certain claims can be made without clinical trials or scientific evidence to support the claims. Therefore, you should be aware of what you're buying and do some research in advance. The ConsumerLab Web site (*www.consumerlab.com*) provides an excellent resource for the contents of many products containing vitamins, minerals, herbals, and dietary supplements. The ConsumerLab site reports the results of independent testing to evaluate manufacturers' claims and the presence of amounts of ingredients in the tested products.

Rimostil (see Question 54) is an isoflavone preparation intended to improve bone density. It is sold in stores and over the Internet. Rimostil is manufactured by Novogen, a pharmaceutical company. There is some evidence that isoflavones from red clover can increase bone density. Novogen's other red clover isoflavone product is Promensil™. Some women say that Promensil gives them relief from hot flashes.

There has been little long-term testing of phytoestrogens such as the isoflavones found in red clover; however, some short-term small studies indicate that they may have a place in improving bone health. If you are looking for a nonprescription way of trying to improve bone density, Rimostil or Promensil may be options for you. However, you should discuss this choice with your clinician. Because Rimostil is made from isoflavones, which are phytoestrogens, it's important to remember that the contraindications to estrogen apply to Rimostil and Promensil as well (history or presence of breast cancer, estrogen-dependent cancers, history of clots, unexplained uterine bleeding). You also need to be aware that these products may not mix well with prescription medications for bone health such as Evista or estrogens.

OsteoSine®, manufactured by NuLiv and taken as two capsules per day, contains vitamins, minerals, and a blend of ingredients made from cuscuta chinensis, an herb that contains flavonoids (the substances in red wine that are believed to contribute to reducing the risk of heart disease). The manufacturer of OsteoSine claims bone health can be improved, but this has not been tested in large clinical trials. To the extent that OsteoSine does contain vitamins and minerals necessary to support good bone health, its claims could be true. Should you decide to go this route, be wary of any unusual rashes or reactions, which may indicate that you are allergic to one of the ingredients that are not specifically named on the label. And as always, make sure that your clinician is aware of any OTC medication you are taking.

Calcium and vitamin D, the most important mineral and vitamin for promoting bone health, are the most accessible OTC treatments and preventive measures for osteoporosis. Don't forget that even if you take adequate amounts of both and exercise properly, you still may not avoid bone loss, especially if you are a woman at or past menopause (see Questions 46–51).

69. How long will I be treated for osteoporosis? How will I know if the treatments are working?

Osteoporosis is beginning to get the scrutiny and concern that it deserves. Up to now, osteoporosis has received little attention, possibly because it causes no pain unless you break a bone or possibly because many people associate it with normal aging. Few therapies for osteoporosis have been tested for use for longer than 10 years, except estrogen, which was approved for

Treatment for primary osteoporosis is usually ongoing unless some contraindications to treatment arise.

the prevention of postmenopausal osteoporosis in 1972. Despite this, treatment for primary osteoporosis is usually ongoing unless some contraindications to treatment arise. In the case of secondary osteoporosis, treatment continues until the secondary cause of osteoporosis is remedied or the medication causing osteoporosis is discontinued and bone density testing reveals stable bone mass over time.

The National Osteoporosis Foundation (NOF) recommends repeat BMD testing to monitor bone loss every 2 years. If you are taking medication therapy, the NOF recommends you be tested again 2 years after starting medication and about every 2 years after that. If you are using lifestyle measures alone to prevent bone loss, the NOF also recommends testing about every 2 years for you. The NOF recommends testing for anyone at risk and for those who would start treatment if they knew they had bone loss.

If you have glucocorticoid-induced osteoporosis (GIO) (see Question 15), the Surgeon General recommends retesting every 6 months until bone mass levels are stable. In all cases of monitoring, DXA testing of the hip and/or spine is the most accurate. Peripheral testing (heel or wrist) is not valuable in the assessment of your progress or for diagnosis of osteoporosis. Although some clinicians may use urinary or blood biomarkers to evaluate whether a certain treatment is working, these markers are not currently predictive of the way patients will respond to treatments. Further study is needed to determine which markers clearly indicate whether BMD is increasing and which markers indicate that fracture risk is reduced (see Question 39).

Depending on the type of medication you are on, the extent of bone loss when you were first tested, and how you are tested for improvement will give you some clues as to the length of your treatment and how often you need to be monitored:

Menopause hormone therapy (MHT). If you are on any product containing estrogen, you will need to be reevaluated at least annually to determine if you should stay on it. Typically, if you are on MHT for hot flashes and night sweats or vaginal dryness, your bones are going to benefit from the estrogen regardless of how long you are on it. Based on the WHI results, most clinicians recommend that estrogen or estrogen-containing products be taken for the shortest period of time possible, usually 5 years or less. After that time, it's believed that the risks of breast cancer and stroke go up enough to outweigh the benefits of estrogen. However, that is a decision to be made by you and your clinician. The fastest rate of bone loss occurs in the first 4 to 8 years following menopause, so if you are on MHT for menopausal symptoms, of course you will benefit from its protective effects on bone. Evidence shows that once MHT is stopped, bone loss increases almost immediately, usually at the same rate as before you started MHT. However, one study found that beneficial effects on bone were present several years later among women who had used MHT in the first 2 to 3 years after menopause. Having regular BMD tests will assist you in your decision-making from the standpoint that if you no longer need MHT for moderate to severe menopausal symptoms, you may need another medication if your DXA test shows osteopenia or osteoporosis.

The fastest rate of bone loss occurs in the first 4 to 8 years following menopause.

Bisphosphonates. Fosamax's (alendronate's) safety record is a good one. So far, Fosamax has been tested for up to 10 years of use without significant problems. Once stopped, Fosamax continues its positive effect on bone mass if you had 5 years of continuous treatment. The other bisphosphonates have also been shown to continue their protective effect after the medication is stopped, but studies have been smaller and for shorter duration than those done using Fosamax. Once you are diagnosed with osteopenia or osteoporosis and placed on a medication, in this case a bisphosphonate, you will not know if it's working unless your BMD test is repeated. Your clinician should tell you when you need to be retested. In most cases, you will be retested about 2 years after you begin treatment. According to the American Association of Clinical Endocrinologists (AACE), you should not stop treatment even if there is no improvement or even a slight decrease in BMD after 2 years of treatment. This makes sense when you consider that an increase of 3% to 6% at the hip or 2% to 4% at the spine is needed to be considered a clinical improvement. Differences in testing machines and testers can account for as much as 5% of the change in measurements. Failure to increase or minimally improve bone density is not a reason to stop or change treatment. Usually, treatment with a bisphosphonate is long term, meaning years.

Evista. Evista (raloxifene) was the first estrogen agonist/antagonist to be approved for the treatment of osteoporosis, and its approval depended on many years of testing for safety. While you are on Evista, BMD testing should follow the usual guidelines for testing about every 2 years. Most of the clinical trials based their results on 3 to 4 years of treatment and established an acceptable safety level during those trials to achieve FDA approval for use. So, while it is not clear at this time how long Evista can be taken, it appears safe for at least 4 years. But remember, once you stop taking it, your bone mass will start to decrease again.

Calcitonin preparations. Miacalcin NS and Fortical (calcitonin) are usually reserved for women who are at least 5 years postmenopause and in whom estrogen therapy is not advised or desired, but they can be used in combination with MHT. Miacalcin NS or Fortical are usually prescribed following a vertebral fracture and most often for pain relief. The effects of calcitonin nasal spray can be monitored by DXA retesting. After 2 years of treatment, there generally is no further increase in bone mass. Although there are no specific standards for monitoring due to the very small changes in bone density that occur with calcitonin preparations, those using calcitonin nasal spray should be monitored about every 2 years. Urinary markers as indicators of improved BMD have not been tested in women using calcitonin nasal spray.

Forteo. Although measurements of BMD were taken after only 3 months in Forteo study participants, your clinician may want to monitor your progress after 1 year of treatment. Using Forteo for longer than 2 years is not recommended because the long-term safety of its use has not been established. A 10-year study of Forteo is under way because the FDA has required a "black-box warning" advising that Forteo may cause a rare form of bone cancer. Your clinician may advise more frequent monitoring of your bones until the results of the 10-year study are known.

Before you leave your clinician's office with a prescription, be sure to find out the expectations in terms of retesting and monitoring your progress.

70. I have early menopause. What does this mean for my bones, and will I need treatment?

Whether your early menopause (also called **premature menopause**) is caused by surgery, is for unknown reasons, or is because of cancer treatments, your bones are at risk and you may need treatment.

When you are trying to cope with the treatments for cancer, it's hard to think about your bones and the possibility of developing osteoporosis so early in life. But the fact is that when you stop having your menstrual periods for whatever reason, your risk of bone loss increases. When you experience a natural menopause around the average age of 51, you can expect to lose bone most rapidly in the 4 to 8 years following menopause (starting 1 year after your last period). There are several reasons why you might experience menopause much earlier than that, and therefore need to cope with a larger stretch of your life without estrogen, an important hormone for bone growth.

A very small percentage of women (1%) experience natural menopause before the age of 40. It is not known why these women stop having their periods. **Idiopathic ovarian insufficiency** or **premature ovarian failure** is a condition that usually occurs in women under the age of 40 and causes menopause. Idiopathic ovarian insufficiency is usually caused by autoimmune and genetic disorders, Addison's disease (disorder of the adrenal glands, which manufacture steroid hormones), or hypothyroidism (an underactive thyroid gland).

Induced menopause is permanent menopause that occurs in women before their natural menopause. It

Premature menopause

Permanent (usually natural) menopause occurring in women younger than 40 years of age; also refers to women who have induced or surgical menopause.

Idiopathic ovarian insufficiency

The loss of ovarian function (and therefore fertility) in a woman under the age of 40, resulting in menopause. It is usually associated with other health conditions, and can sometimes be temporary. Also called premature ovarian failure.

Induced menopause

Permanent menopause that is not natural; can be caused as a result of surgical removal of the ovaries, chemotherapy, or radiation to the pelvis.

occurs when the ovaries are removed along with the uterus and fallopian tubes (often called a **total hysterectomy**; the technical term is total hysterectomy with bilateral **salpingo-oophorectomy**). Once the ovaries are removed, menopause is sudden and the accompanying symptoms of hot flashes, sleep disruptions, and mood changes can be quite severe. The ovaries no longer can secrete estrogen, and bone loss may start to occur almost immediately as well.

If only the uterus is removed, menopause occurs earlier than usual but not abruptly. An earlier menopause is believed to result from the decreased blood supply to the ovaries, which can occur after surgery to remove only the uterus. Many people have the misconception that if the uterus is removed, a woman goes into menopause. However, she only stops having menstrual periods; her ovaries continue to make estrogen. The estrogen will continue to have a protective effect on her bones until her ovaries stop producing estrogen, most likely earlier than the average age of 51. However, she will not be able to gauge exactly when menopause actually occurs because she will not have the usual cessation of her menses for 12 months, the hallmark of menopause.

Surgically induced menopause (removal of both ovaries) will cause you to lose bone fairly rapidly. It is important for you to prevent bone loss by getting the appropriate amounts of calcium (1200 to 1500 mg), vitamin D (400 to 800 IU), other necessary nutrients (see Table 6 in Question 53), and exercise. You should also be sure to make lifestyle changes that could improve your bone health, like avoiding heavy alcohol use and stopping smoking. In addition, you and your clinician may want to discuss medications

Total hysterectomy

Although technically only refers to removal of the uterus, "total" is sometimes used to refer to removal of the uterus, ovaries, and fallopian tubes.

Salpingo-oophorectomy

Removal of fallopian tube and ovary; *bilateral* means both fallopian tubes and both ovaries are removed.

Lifestyle Changes and Treatments

for preventing bone loss. As long as your surgery did not result from cancer and you do not have any contraindications to taking them, you may take any of the medications that are approved for prevention of osteoporosis. If you are experiencing significant symptoms resulting from your induced menopause, a good option for you may be MHT (see Questions 64 and 66). Your clinician may also want to send you for BMD testing to get a baseline reading of your bones.

Induced menopause can also be a result of chemotherapy and radiation used to treat cancers. While surgically induced menopause always causes an abrupt stoppage of the production of estrogen by the ovary, chemotherapy and radiation to the pelvis stops ovarian secretion of estrogen, but sometimes this occurs over a longer period of time. This often means that women undergoing radiation and chemotherapy will have more time to adjust to the loss of estrogen. But it also means that they will begin to lose bone once the ovaries have stopped making hormones.

While women who have their ovaries removed for reasons unrelated to cancer could use MHT to treat their symptoms and to prevent osteoporosis, breast cancer survivors will have fewer options to treat their symptoms and to prevent bone loss. Few women who experience breast cancer can take estrogen because many cancers are linked to estrogen or are dependent on them for their growth (termed estrogen dependent or **estrogen receptor positive cancer**). After treatment, some women with estrogen receptor positive cancer will be prescribed tamoxifen, an estrogen agonist/antagonist, to prevent a recurrence of breast cancer. Tamoxifen is known to increase bone mineral density in the spine by

Estrogen receptor positive cancer

Type of cancer that is estrogen dependent or has receptors for estrogen.

about 1% per year, but it causes bone loss in women who are healthy and premenopausal even though it increases BMD in healthy postmenopausal women. Nolvadex (tamoxifen) is not currently approved for the prevention or treatment of osteoporosis. Evista (raloxifene), another estrogen agonist/antagonist, is an option for breast cancer survivors if they are postmenopausal. Evista is FDA-approved for preventing invasive breast cancer in postmenopausal women with osteoporosis, or women who are at increased risk for invasive breast cancer. Evista is also approved for the prevention and treatment of postmenopausal osteoporosis (see Question 61).

Women whose breast cancers are not estrogen receptor positive generally are not treated with an estrogen agonist/antagonist. And most clinicians will not prescribe MHT to breast cancer patients even if the cancer is not estrogen dependent. Regardless of the type of breast cancer, any woman with chemotherapy-induced menopause will be at risk for losing bone. If you have a test that shows osteoporosis, your treatment options include the bisphosphonates, Evista, and calcitonin (see Questions 56–59, 61, and 63). Because many tumor cells secrete a substance related to parathyroid hormone, it is not clear if Forteo (teriparatide, a synthetic parathyroid hormone) would be an option for treatment in breast cancer survivors. Other treatment options are under study. For example, the bisphosphonate Zometa (zoledronate) is being evaluated for osteoporosis treatment in breast cancer survivors. So far, there is strong evidence that the bone density of the women taking Zometa has increased, but further study is needed to confirm the improvement and to document the long-term effects. Several options are also available to prevent osteoporosis in women who have had chemotherapy, such as the bisphosphonates and estrogen agonists/antagonists as well as lifestyle changes that include calcium supplementation, vitamin D, exercise, diet modifications, and smoking cessation.

Chemotherapy or pelvic radiation used to treat cancer can also induce menopause and the bone loss that follows the loss of estrogen. Although men don't experience menopause, they can have significant bone loss and fragility fractures when treated with GnRH agonists for prostate cancer. GnRH agonists such as Lupron are also used to treat endometriosis in women. Bone loss is one of the major side effects of Lupron.

Advanced breast cancer, advanced prostate cancer, and a cancer called multiple myeloma are all associated with bone metastases. The spread of cancer cells to the bone causes loss of strength of the bone, significant pain, and an increased risk of fracture. So those with cancer can have considerable bone loss and a significant increase in fractures, which result from the treatments for the cancer and the spread of the cancer itself.

Complementary therapies

Therapies that are used in addition to conventional, Western medical treatments or interventions.

Alternative therapies

Therapies that are used in place of conventional Western medical therapies; includes massage, visualization, naturopathic medicine, and acupuncture, among others.

71. Are there any complementary or alternative therapies that are effective for osteoporosis or osteopenia? Can I have a massage, or will that hurt my bones?

Complementary therapies are therapies that are used in addition to conventional (sometimes called "Western") medical treatments or interventions. **Alternative therapies** are therapies that are used in place of conventional medical treatments. The use of these therapies has increased dramatically over the years. In fact, a recent study of Americans found that when prayer is included as a complementary and alternative medicine (CAM) therapy, 62% of Americans used CAM therapies in the preceding 12 months. But large clinical studies that compare a CAM therapy with a placebo or with a conventional treatment have rarely been funded, so making a case in support of using CAM therapies to prevent or treat osteoporosis is difficult.

The National Center for Complementary and Alternative Medicine (NCCAM), a division of the National Institutes of Health, divides CAM into the following categories:

- Alternative medical systems such as acupuncture and naturopathic medicine
- Mind–body interventions such as prayer and guided imagery
- Biologically based therapies such as dietary supplements and phytoestrogens
- Manipulative therapies such as acupressure and massage
- Energy-based therapies such as magnet therapy and therapeutic touch

Practitioners of chiropractic, the CAM practice that involves manipulating and aligning bones and surrounding tissues correctly, are educated about ways to modify manipulation techniques to avoid fractures of weak bones. Some chiropractors do not manipulate or align any bones in patients with osteoporosis. They may prefer instead to play a teaching role in counseling patients about appropriate calcium and vitamin D intake, healthy diet, and particularly how to avoid fracturing their bones when exercising. They may also help patients to learn appropriate strengthening exercises, targeting specific muscles.

In some studies of acupuncture, results have been mixed. For the treatment of osteoporosis, acupuncture is more commonly used with herbs in the practice of traditional Chinese medicine (TCM). According to TCM, the kidneys govern the bones, so TCM therapies target strengthening the kidney. Herbs that may be used to treat or prevent osteoporosis include those that boost estrogen levels, such as black cohosh, cypress, sage, ginseng, and licorice, and those that enhance mineral use by the body, such as horsetail, stinging nettle, and knotweed. Before using herbs to prevent or treat osteoporosis, you should consult your clinician and a licensed herbalist. Many of these herbs can interact or interfere with your existing medications.

While not all of the CAM therapies would be appropriate for the management or prevention of osteoporosis, some therapies may help in the management of pain from fractures. For example, hypnotherapy and guided imagery might be helpful. When pain causes stress, there are a number of CAM therapies that would be appropriate for stress management, including massage, aromatherapy, mindfulness, and yoga, to name a few (see Question 82).

Massage is gaining popularity not only because it is relaxing, but because many in the massage field believe that human touch can help all conditions. Massage has been shown to improve pain levels, particularly in people with arthritis, cancer, and low back pain. Most practitioners of massage will take a history from you, and you should be sure to mention that you have osteoporosis if you're not asked specifically. If you are having a chair massage, it is important to refrain from bending your spine forward, as this potentially may cause compression fractures of your spine.

Massages while you're lying down are definitely appropriate and can be beneficial to your stress level. Because it can ease the pain associated with many conditions, massage is a useful adjunct to self-healing. Some believe that massage can help to increase bone mass, at least indirectly, because it can relieve pain, which in turn can make exercise more manageable, and because it can help muscles become more flexible, making exercise more effective for bone health. If they are made aware of any vertebral fractures, massage therapists will be careful to avoid directly manipulating the tissue near the bones in the back. Massage increases blood flow to all areas of the body, improving your circulation, which can boost healing and reduce pain.

Lifestyle Changes and Treatments

PART FOUR

Living with Osteoporosis

Which bones am I more likely to break?

I always hear about older folks fracturing hips. Is this because of osteoporosis or because of the frequency of falls? How are broken hips repaired?

It's hard not to think about my bones being weak. How do I keep osteoporosis from interfering with my life?

More...

72. Will the treatments help me make new bone, or will there always be holes? Will I be more likely to break a bone? Does a fracture look differently on a bone with osteoporosis?

Though many people think that we're done making new bone after we reach young adulthood, bone is an active and dynamic tissue throughout our lives. The process of bone breakdown and new bone formation is always going on. Of course, it does slow down as we approach the end of life. Osteoporosis treatment and prevention strategies are intended to slow down bone breakdown and speed up bone formation. If you are on Actonel (risedronate), Fosamax (alendronate), Boniva (ibandronate), Reclast (zoledronic acid), Miacalcin NS (calcitonin), Fortical (calcitonin), Evista (raloxifene), or MHT (estrogen, progestin), your treatments are targeting the osteoclasts, the cells that break down bone. If you are taking Forteo (teriparatide), your treatment helps your body build new bone, rather than just slowing down the process of bone breakdown. Don't forget that there are two characteristics about bone that put you at greater risk for fracture. Bone mineral density together with the quality of the bone determine how strong your bones are and how easily they can break. So, you can increase your bone density, but you may still be at considerable risk for breaking a bone.

Bone mineral density together with the quality of the bone determine how strong your bones are and how easily they can break.

Depending on the balance in the bone breakdown–formation cycle, you have the potential to reduce those holes left by the osteoclasts. If your treatments help the osteoblasts form more bone than the osteoclasts break down, you will make new bone. The new bone will improve your bone density T-score when you are retested after treatments. In order for the increased bone mass to be clinically significant on the DXA testing, your bone mass will need to have increased by more than 2% to 4% at the spine and 3% to 6% at the hip. If you stop your treatment, the cycle of remodeling bone will likely once again favor bone breakdown, and holes will reappear. The positive effects of some of the medications remain even after the medication has been stopped. This is another important consideration in the medication you select with your clinician.

If you are being treated for bone loss, you are still more likely to break a bone even though you are on medication, because for each standard deviation that your score is below zero, your fracture risk increases. But numbers are not what matter most here. Being aware that you can break a bone more easily if you fall should prompt you to make changes in your environment to prevent falling. Question 79 has some tips about preventing falls. It should also help you to remember your medication. Taking your medication exactly as it is prescribed is very important to improving your bone health.

Being aware that you can break a bone more easily if you fall should prompt you to make changes in your environment to prevent falling.

In order for osteoporosis to become apparent on a conventional x-ray, you would have lost 30% to 40% of your bone mass. But even though lower bone mass can be seen on x-rays, osteoporosis is not diagnosed by those x-rays, and DXA testing is still needed (see Question 23). Conversely, fractures can be read on conventional x-rays and do not require DXA imaging for diagnosis. Some fractures, like vertebral compression fractures, can be difficult to diagnose even by conventional x-rays, so additional testing may be needed. Fractures that occur with very little force or trauma are most likely related to osteoporosis. Conventional x-rays show the entire bone rather than focusing on density, and osteoporosis does not interfere with identifying a fracture. It's the fracture itself and especially the way the fracture occurred that might make your clinician suspicious of osteoporosis, if you have not already been diagnosed with it (see Question 74).

73. Which bones am I more likely to break?

For all women with or without osteoporosis who are 50 years or older, the lifetime risk of fracturing any bone is about 40%, though most fractures occurring after age 50 are related to osteoporosis. For all U.S. adults, the lifetime risk of fracturing a bone is greater than the combined risk of developing breast, uterine, or ovarian cancers. If you are a woman, the risk of fracturing your hip, your spine, or your wrist is between 15% and 18% each. If you are a White older woman who either has hyperthyroidism (overactive thyroid), cannot get out of a chair without using your arms, or has a resting pulse rate of over 80 beats per minute, the risk for fracturing your hip is about 70%. If your only risk factor is that your mother broke her hip, then your risk is about 80%, but it's only about 50% if you fractured any of your bones since the age of 50. Even without any of these specific risk factors, age increases your risk for fracture by about 40% every 5 years. Your risk for hip fracture increases with more risk factors, so making changes to reduce your risk, such as increasing exercise, getting enough vitamin D and calcium, and quitting smoking, is important. The FRAX algorithm makes it possible to determine your individual 10-year risk probability for a hip fracture and for any major osteoporotic fracture (see Question 55).

There are more fractures related to osteoporosis than the combined number of heart attacks, strokes, and new diagnoses of breast cancer among women each year.

All together, there are more fractures related to osteoporosis than the combined number of heart attacks, strokes, and new diagnoses of breast cancer among women each year. The combined 250,000 hip fractures,

250,000 wrist fractures, 750,000 spinal fractures, and 250,000 other fractures amounts to 1.5 million fractures related to osteoporosis per year. So, if you are going to break a bone, you are about 3 times more likely to break a bone in your spine than you are in your hip. And you are just as likely to break your wrist as your hip.

Marie's comment:

My grandmother had osteoporosis. Well, actually, I don't think she was ever officially diagnosed with it, but she must have had it because she had so many broken bones. I remember when she visited us at our house when she was about 85 or 86 and she had such terrible back pain, she couldn't even get dressed by herself. She told us she had fallen onto her bottom and back when she was at home and reached up into her closet to get something off the top shelf. She didn't fall that far or hard, but she said her back had been hurting ever since. We took her to the doctor and they did x-rays that showed she had 4 or 5 fractures in her spine bones. She was admitted to the hospital and was progressing slowly, and then she came home to our house and recuperated there for another 2 or 3 weeks. She eventually went back to her home (after about 2 months all together), but within 2 weeks she fell again, this time in the bathtub, and was admitted to the hospital. This time she had cracked her pelvis and was eventually admitted to a nursing home. After she had been in the nursing home for 6 years or so, she broke her thigh bone while trying to get out of bed. Her leg got caught up in the side rail on the bed, and when she turned, it just broke. She wasn't ever treated for osteoporosis, except for taking calcium. And she wasn't at such high risk. She was a good-sized woman, not fat or anything, but not frail. And she was active her whole life. But after she cracked her pelvis, she never left that nursing home. She died there.

74. I am 45 years old. I recently stumbled on a rug. I fell against the wall. I broke my wrist and my clinician is now concerned that I have osteoporosis. She called my fracture a "fragility fracture." What is that, and what does it have to do with osteoporosis?

Fragility fracture

Term used to describe fractures that occur with very little trauma or force and from a height that is usually not great enough to cause broken bones, usually indicating that the bone is weak. Also called osteoporotic fractures.

Fragility fracture is a term used by clinicians to describe fractures that occur without much force and from a height usually not great enough to cause broken bones. They are also called osteoporotic fractures. The term is used to help clinicians evaluate the state of their patients' bones. A history or presence of one or more fragility fractures also helps clinicians in the decision to send you for BMD testing and treat you for osteoporosis (see Questions 19 and 20). The degree of osteoporosis is also diagnosed by the presence or history of fragility fractures. Severe osteoporosis is diagnosed when BMD indicates a T-score more than 2.5 standard deviations below the mean with a history or presence of one or more fragility fractures. However, you don't have to have osteoporosis to have a fragility fracture. In fact, according to the NORA (National Osteoporosis Risk Assessment) study, 50% of fragility fractures occur in individuals with osteopenia. Interestingly enough, you can even have a fragility fracture while still having normal BMD.

One of the problems with fragility fractures is that sometimes they occur not because you have osteoporosis or low bone mass as measured by BMD testing, but because your bones have poor bone quality. This means that while your bone density tests may indicate that you have normal bone density, the "architecture" of the bones may be weak. Machines used to measure BMD cannot "see" inside the bone to evaluate its structure, and therefore a DXA machine cannot measure your bone quality. Because BMD testing does not measure bone quality, your risk of getting a fragility fracture may still be high despite a normal T-score.

Because most of the research has been conducted on women over the age of 65, there are not enough data yet to provide useful information on younger women and men. So, even though younger women are not expected to be at high risk for fracture, your clinician is right to be concerned simply based on the low level of force of your fall. Some clinicians believe that the angle of breaking a bone determines whether the bone has enough strength to withstand force. This would be likened to a breakable dish that when dropped at one angle may shatter, but from another angle it remains unharmed. Your bone strength could actually be quite weak even though your bones appear to be normal on BMD testing.

Fragility fractures can happen when you fall or bang against something, but most often they occur spontaneously in your back (see Question 83). Sometimes you will experience significant pain with a vertebral fracture and other times it will be "silent," meaning that a fracture occurs but you are not even aware of it.

If you experience a fragility fracture, your clinician will send you for a DXA test. You also will be evaluated for possible causes, such as using medication that weakens bones or having an illness that interferes with bone development or quality (see Questions 15 and 16).

If possible secondary causes for the fragility fracture are ruled out, you should be referred to a specialist to discuss treatment for osteoporosis. This presents an opportunity for beginning medications for osteoporosis to increase bone density and to decrease further fracture risk, even though the quality of your bones may cause you to fracture a bone more easily. You should also receive counseling about your calcium and vitamin D intake, exercise, and any lifestyle changes that may improve the health of your bones. Once you have sustained one fracture, you are at high risk for having another, so it's important to evaluate your surroundings for the things that could put you at risk for falling. Question 79 discusses ways to reduce your risk of falls. You would also want to make sure that you are not bending forward or twisting your spine if you have bone loss in the spine, since both actions could cause vertebral fractures. Figure 10 in Question 44 shows exercises to avoid.

75. If I fracture a bone, will it change my treatment? Will a broken bone take longer to heal? Will a broken bone be repaired or casted differently?

To heal a broken bone can be challenging at any age, but if you have osteoporosis, you are more likely to be in your middle years or older. Healing does happen more slowly as we age. It is more important than ever that you have a healthy diet and get the proper nutrients for healing. Your diet should be a healthy one, including adequate but not excessive protein. You should also be especially careful to get the appropriate amounts of vitamins and minerals, particularly calcium and vitamins A, C, and D, all of which contribute to healthy bone development and healing whether you have a fracture or not. You should stay on your osteoporosis medication unless told otherwise by your clinician, but it's also a good idea to ask if there are any medications you should discontinue while you are healing.

Depending on which bone you break, the repair and treatment may be a little different:

Hip. Because you will be less mobile for a period of time (see Questions 77 and 78), it is important for you to stop certain medications that can put you at risk for blood clots, such as Evista (raloxifene) and MHT (estrogen or estrogen and progesterone). Casts are not applied to broken hips the way they are for other broken bones. Broken hips can take a very long time to heal, and complete healing may never take place. Many factors contribute to the healing process, not the least of which is the person's physical condition prior to the broken hip. The caretakers, who themselves may be quite a bit older, may not be able to provide the intensive care that is often needed for recovery. And the isolation associated with immobility can lead to severe depression, which has a huge impact on healing.

Wrist. Fracturing a bone in your forearm, usually near your wrist, does not cause the same problems of disability and even death that are attributed to hip fractures. However, wrist fractures can cause persistent pain, functional and nerve problems, bone deformities, and arthritis. Although a wrist fracture is less likely to cause problems with walking and being mobile, it can still restrict you from getting out of the house, especially if you need to drive. It can also prevent you from doing activities of daily living, such as bathing and meal preparation. You will likely have a cast applied to your forearm, which includes the area below the elbow down to the thumb and fingers. Typically, a simple fracture requires a cast for 4 to 6 weeks, but depending on your ability to heal, you may have a cast longer.

Vertebral fractures. Fractures of the spine can be painful or they can be "silent," meaning that they are present but not necessarily painful (see Question 83). These types of fractures cannot be put in a cast. However, some clinicians might still recommend that you wear a metal brace that prevents your spine from twisting or bending. There is controversy about whether a brace provides sufficient pain relief to warrant its use and whether the immobility provided by the brace causes more harm than good, so braces are recommended infrequently. Vertebral fractures can cause considerable disability and distress. In addition to staying on your currently prescribed medication, Miacalcin NS or Fortical may be added to ease some of the pain associated with your spine fractures, and it may work with your current medication to increase your bone density even further. This type of fracture can take many weeks to heal. Unfortunately, simply having one osteoporotic spinal fracture significantly increases your risk of having another within 1 year's time.

Roxanne's comment:

Although my ankle fracture occurred about 5 months ago, I think it's going to take me a full year to recover. I never would have guessed that this type of fracture could take so long to heal. I still have some pain and quite a lot of swelling, although I'm able to get around on my own. My orthopedist said that I should expect to have arthritis in the ankle and to go back to the elliptical machine instead of walking as my form of exercise. I have started taking estrogen again for my menopause symptoms, although I had stopped it during my recovery because I was fairly immobile.

When I first fractured my ankle, the surgeon came out with crutches, expecting me to use them. He obviously didn't know I was a klutz and would have broken the other ankle if I actually continued to use them. I constantly felt like I was going to fall. Crutches and walkers are the equivalent of walking on your hands! So, instead of seeing a wheelchair as a sign of failure, I saw it as my only option to get around. I went everywhere in it. That wheelchair allowed me to go back to work and to do almost everything I was used to doing before the accident. I used nothing but a wheelchair at home, too. I was home alone during the day for about a month, and I was petrified of falling while using crutches or a walker. The wheelchair was the single most important reason I was able to stay active and mobile. And it saved me both financially and socially because I was able to return to work probably about 6 weeks sooner than I would have had I stayed on crutches. I tell everyone that a wheelchair is not a sign of weakness or failure!

Recovering from a fracture like this has been an enlightening experience for me. I look for handrails and handicapped access everywhere I go now. I never realized how seriously breaking a bone could impact your life. I'm very conscious now of not putting myself in situations where I could fall. Although I was wearing low-heeled, rubber-soled shoes when I fell, I recommend wearing high-top sneakers and cowboy boots for their ankle support!

76. My clinician told me not to take up skiing or ice-skating now that I have bone loss. Why is that, and are there other activities I should avoid?

High-impact winter sports are discouraged for people who have any degree of bone loss unless you have always been a skier or skater. The learning curve for these types of sports involves many falls, which is the reason to avoid them. The impact from the falls further increases your risk for a fracture. Even professional skiers and skaters fall sometimes. It has nothing to do with stamina or willingness to learn. It has to do with the likelihood of falling. Any sport that involves a high possibility for falls should be avoided.

And it's not just winter sports. For example, if you've never run the 100-meter high hurdles or done horseback riding, now is not the time to start! Similarly, you should avoid sports that are high impact, where there is a strong possibility that you will have rough contact or be knocked over by another player. So, sports such as football, soccer, field hockey, softball, and kick-boxing are best avoided if you have osteoporosis.

Midlife and beyond, particularly if you are retired, present many opportunities to try new things and explore your interests. It's great to take up the challenge of learning and trying new things! Remaining physically active is very important, but stick to new activities that have low impact and low risk for falls.

If you have been told that you have osteoporosis or if you have a history of spinal fractures, it is particularly important to avoid forward bending or twisting of your spine. You should be careful to avoid toe touches, sit-ups, and some movements in yoga and Tai chi (see Questions 43 and 44). If you have been told that you have osteopenia (T-score of −1.0 to −2.5), you can still do exercises that involve forward bending or twisting of the spine as long as the bone loss is not in your spine (see Figure 10 in Question 44).

77. Should I stop exercising if I break a bone?

Exercise and physical activity are so important to your overall health and well-being that the simple answer is "no." However, if you break your hip, then your legs will be immobilized before surgery and immediately afterward (see Question 78). Probably you will be encouraged to move your upper body, and you may need to shift in bed using a "trapeze" over your head. Even though you may not be using a walker immediately, you need to retain your upper body strength so that when you do get moving, you will be strong enough to support yourself. One of the reasons that it's so important to keep a well-conditioned upper body is that you never know when you may need to rely on your arms to help you move around.

A broken wrist will prevent you from doing many activities, but regular exercise doesn't need to be one of them. Obviously, you can't swim or lift weights with the affected arm. However, walking, stationary biking, and other activities that don't require the use of your arm can keep you in good physical shape. A cast can cause poor balance, making it more likely that you will fall. So, running and any sport that requires running would be best to avoid until your wrist is completely healed.

If you break a bone in your spine, you will probably not be able to continue your regular exercise routine, particularly if you need to wear a back brace. If you are accustomed to walking or other weight-bearing exercise, you should continue to walk, but instead of 30 minutes at a time, try a few minutes per hour. Sitting for long periods without movement can actually cause more pain and stiffness. Be very aware of your posture as you sit and walk, and keep your head up and your spine straight. Keeping your shoulders back and your abdominal muscles pulled in will also increase your back muscle strength to support your spine. You can do some gentle arm and shoulder exercises when you are sitting, but use pain as your guide. If just lifting a teacup causes pain, then activities using the arms and shoulders may need to be avoided for a while. Some experts suggest partial squat exercises, which help to increase the strength of your thigh muscles, without causing additional stress on the spine.

78. I always hear about older folks fracturing their hips. Is this because of osteoporosis or because of the frequency of falls? How are broken hips repaired?

Almost 350,000 people are hospitalized for hip fractures in the United States every year, and most of them are women over the age of 65. White women are hospitalized for hip fracture at a rate five times that of Black women. However, Black women have more disability and death related to their fractures than White women. If you are a Black woman, you are 2 to 3 times more likely to die from a hip fracture than your White counterpart.

Because 95% of hip fractures occur as a result of falls, it is important to look at ways of preventing them (see Question 79). Breaking a hip may be the first sign that someone has osteoporosis. If you have already lost 30% to 40% of the bone in your hip, then bone loss may be visible on the x-ray. If your hip fracture occurs from a low level of trauma (like falling out of bed), you may be diagnosed with osteoporosis without having a bone

Breaking a hip may be the first sign that someone has osteoporosis.

density test done. If not, then you may not be officially diagnosed with osteoporosis until a BMD test confirms it, although it's unlikely that BMD testing would be done while you're in the hospital. As part of your hip fracture management, you may be placed on a medication to treat osteoporosis (see Question 74).

If you fall, the signs and symptoms that you may have a hip fracture include severe pain in the hip or groin, inability to bear weight, a shortened leg on the side with the potential fracture, and bruising or swelling in the groin. Sometimes the position of your leg (turning inward or outward) after falling or trauma can be a clue for your clinician to the possibility of hip fracture. **Figure 12** shows the normal pelvis, hips, and usual locations of hip fractures.

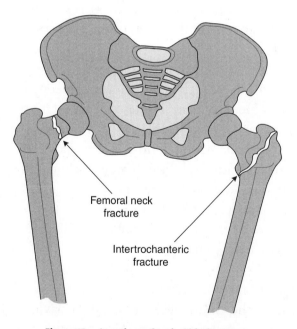

Femoral neck
fracture

Intertrochanteric
fracture

Figure 12   Locations of typical hip fractures.

In people who are likely to have severe complications related to surgery, orthopedic surgeons use a traction (tension) system to help the hip fracture heal. But the extended immobility associated with this treatment has its own complications. Being immobile for a long time can lead to blood clots, urinary incontinence, loss of muscle conditioning, pneumonia, pressure sores (bedsores), depression, social isolation, and greater bone loss. Unfortunately, once you fracture your hip or any other bone, you are at greater risk of fracturing a bone again.

The surgical treatment of your hip fracture will depend on the sites of the fracture. If you fracture the femoral neck (Figure 12), you may have a screw inserted, a partial hip replacement, or a total hip replacement. The total hip replacement involves replacing both the upper part of your femur bone, the "ball" of the bone, and the socket into which the ball fits. If you break the intertrochanteric part of the bone (Figure 12), you are likely to have a special compression screw inserted with a metal plate to keep the edges of the bone together.

The recovery time in the hospital after surgery is usually about 1 week. If you don't have someone to assist you at home, a nursing home or rehabilitation center stay may be required so that you can also get the necessary physical therapy. Hip fractures can cause considerable expense and disability, not to mention social isolation, depression, and even death. As you age, you should make every effort to avoid falls and to strengthen your bones so that if you do fall, you will be less likely to break a bone again.

The physical recovery from hip fractures may take less time than the emotional aftereffects of having a fracture. Fractures can interfere significantly with your independence. The realization that you can no longer do for yourself what you've always done can be devastating. In a study of previously independent adults following hip fractures, two-thirds of them were unable to get on and off the toilet without help 12 months after the fracture, and 83% could not bathe or shower by themselves. No wonder depression can set in! A vicious cycle of fear, isolation, dependence, and depression can result. In the event of a hip fracture in yourself or in a loved one, you should pay attention to the very real possibility of depression.

- Get the medical and nursing care that you need. If the discharge planners at the hospital where you have been cared for do not provide you with home care, have a relative arrange it for you. Many insurance plans will provide for visiting nurses and health aides in place of paying for extended hospitalizations. Medicare will also pay, at least partially, for these types of services. In many cases, you may need to go from the hospital to a rehabilitation hospital. If you don't seem to be making progress, ask for a reevaluation.
- Allow family and friends to help you. It may seem rather ironic that in order to keep your independence in the long term, you may need to ask for some help in the short term. Let people help you—giving others the opportunity to help you may also help allay their sense of helplessness about your situation and make them feel needed.
- Family and friends may not know about your hip fracture. Contact friends and family to let them know you may need some assistance in the days and weeks following surgery. Sometimes even if they know, they won't contact you for fear of disturbing you. Let them know about your surgery and that you

would appreciate their support. If they ask what you need, be specific, even if it's only to check on you by phone once a week. If people bring lots of food, ask someone to help you organize smaller meals.

- If you are accustomed to a particular daily activity (e.g., walking with a friend) or weekly activity (such as playing cards), try to stay on your friends' radar screens. Have the friend come to your house and exercise instead of walking. Invite the card-playing friends over for a shorter-than-usual gathering. The main idea is to stay on the calendar and keep in touch.
- Fear of falling or getting another fracture can be intimidating. Be cautious, but don't isolate yourself from going out once you are able. If you're used to driving yourself to church, ask a fellow church member for a ride.
- Just because you are less independent, this doesn't mean you can't use your brain. Continue to stay mentally active. Keep up with the news. Read. Do crossword puzzles. Talk to friends by phone.
- Nip the signs of depression in the bud (see Question 82). Contact your clinician or a mental health professional for help.

Marjory's comment:

I really can understand why people with depression get osteoporosis or why people with osteoporosis get depressed. It's so sad and depressing when you stay home and don't get out and get moving. Exercise doesn't just help you feel better physically and help you sleep better—exercise makes you feel so much better about yourself. It's good for me to get out of the house. Taking classes is such a good thing to do socially. I enjoy being with other people. Occasionally someone will join our water exercise class and might be withdrawn and reluctant to be there for whatever reason. After a few classes when we call each other by name, they really start to enjoy themselves. When I try to do the exercises by myself, I find I don't stick with finishing the exercises, work as hard, or enjoy it nearly as much as I do when I take a class with others. In our area, if you can't drive yourself to exercise classes, there is a bus for seniors that can take you to "health-related" activities, like medical appointments and the pharmacy. I can't think of anything more "health-related" than exercise! Going to a scheduled exercise class gives me some-place specific to go. When I get home, I tell my husband about the people I saw, maybe a joke I heard, and it really gives us something to talk about every day. I have also found that exercising helps me sexually. Sex is so much more comfortable when I'm feeling fit and good about myself. My feeling is that we're all going to have aches and pains, and sometimes it feels easier to stay home and not do anything, but you know what? You're going to have those aches and pains no matter what, so you may as well live well, get out with others, and have a good time.

79. What are some ways to prevent falls?

Because falls account for 95% of bone fractures, it's important to find ways to prevent them. When people fall in their homes, others may wonder how that can happen in a familiar environment. But you can fall anywhere, including your own home where you may have walked the same floors for half of your life. You may have medical conditions that contribute to a loss of balance. You may be rushing to answer the phone or get to the bathroom. Or you may trip on that piece of carpet you've been meaning to tack down for a long time. (**Table 18** lists ways of preventing falls.) There are things you can do now to help you take control and prevent falls. It's not just the new lamp with a long cord that can trip you. If you

Table 18   Preventing Falls

Outdoor Environment	Home Interior	Personal Issues
Remove snow and ice; sand walkways and driveways for better traction.	Do not use scatter or throw type of rugs.	Avoid excessive alcohol.
Install railings near steps.	Tack down loose carpet.	Wear rubber-soled, low-heeled shoes (do not wear backless slip-on shoes or slippers).
Clear clutter from outdoor steps and entryways.	Clear clutter from stairs and rooms.	Do not rush from room to room (e.g., to answer the phone).
Install good lighting.	Move electrical cords and wires out of walking path.	Use cane or walker as needed; don't be afraid to ask for assistance when needed.
If possible, install garage door openers.	Install good lighting in every room.	Use great care when using a step stool.
Keep extra cane or walker in car.	Keep a flashlight next to your bed.	Get appropriate eyeglasses to correct poor vision.
Keep flashlight in the car in case walkways are not well lit.	Use nightlights.	Be aware of your surroundings, e.g., watch for raised thresholds between doorways.
Pay attention to "Caution—Wet Floors" signs and floors that look wet without a sign.	Keep a step stool available to reach things. It should have wide steps and, if possible, a high handrail.	When visiting outside your own home, walk slowly and carefully, watching for obstacles.
Do not walk across uneven surfaces such as gravel driveways.	Install grab bars next to the toilet and in the bathtub/shower.	Use caution when crossing the street.
Stay off grassy slopes, as they can be particularly slippery, especially when wet.	Consider installing a raised toilet seat.	Watch for uneven surfaces, ice, and loose sand.

(cont.)

Table 18 Preventing Falls (*cont.*)

Outdoor Environment	Home Interior	Personal Issues
Get help for yard work or snow removal as needed.	Use a rubber mat that is suctioned to the bathtub or install nonskid surface in tub and shower.	Do not walk at night without good lighting.
	When linoleum and tile floors are washed at home, do not walk on them until they are dry.	Develop strength, flexibility, and balance through exercise.
	Install a bedside phone to call for help in case you feel too unsteady to get out of bed.	Be aware of your risk factors: • Medications that cause dizziness or sedation • Medications that cause diuresis (leading to frequent trips to the bathroom) • Illnesses affecting balance such as stroke, Parkinson's, Alzheimer's, postural hypotension, urinary incontinence, flu • Conditions affecting your feet (e.g., neuropathy of diabetes) • Depression
	Keep a shower chair available to avoid having to sit in the bathtub.	When getting out of bed, rise in stages, sitting first, and getting up slowly.
		Do not wear extra long robes, nightgowns, skirts, or pants.
		Take one step at a time on stairs.

are placed on a new medication or you develop a new symptom such as fever or dehydration, you are more likely to fall. So it's particularly important to be aware of any change in your personal circumstances as well as any changes in your environment.

The more risk factors you have for falling, the more likely you will fall. Risk factors for falling include:

- Age > 65
- Female
- Frailty
- Poor balance or poor vision
- Alzheimer's disease or any condition that impairs thinking or memory, including depression
- Weakness or numbness in the feet or legs
- Medications such as those used to treat depression, psychosis, and high blood pressure
- Medical conditions such as arthritis, vitamin D deficiency, stroke, Parkinson's, infection, dehydration, fever, sudden blood pressure or pulse changes
- Previous fall

While you may not have any control over some of your medical conditions or the medications used to treat them, you do have some control over exercise. Increasing your strength, balance, and coordination can reduce your risk of falling. Tai chi has been shown to reduce the risk of falling in frail older people, reduce the rate of bone loss, and also reduce the number of fractures, possibly due to fewer falls from improved balance. Don't underestimate the importance of the improved balance, coordination, and flexibility that results from exercise.

If you or a family member has many risk factors for falling, you may want to invest in a medical alarm to alert medical and rescue personnel if you or a family member falls. Bed rails are available for non-hospital beds. Getting up in a dark room may make falls more likely. Be sure to have a well-lit path to the bathroom. If you don't want to wake your partner with extra light, keep a small flashlight next to the bed.

If you are on a number of different medications, it's important to make sure that you are taking the correct dosage at the appropriate time every day. Using a pill-minder allows you to stock each compartment with your daily allotment of pills. That makes it less likely that you will take too much of any of your medications, some of which might lower your blood pressure and make you drowsy or dizzy, causing you to fall. You should also avoid the use of alcohol and discuss any over-the-counter medications with your clinician prior to taking them.

80. My clinician has advised that I use hip protectors. What are they, and why should I use them?

Your clinician is concerned that you are at risk for falling. If you do fall, **hip protectors**, which are thick cushioning pads that fit over the hips, may prevent you from fracturing your hip.

Hip protector

A protective pad worn on the hip.

Hip protectors are available in different styles and sizes. Hip pads that fit into washable underwear cushion the blow of a fall, but these pads are not washable. Another style has pads sewn into the underwear in the space over the hips and is fully washable. A third style of protector fits over regular underwear but under your clothes. A belt-type hip guard can be worn outside clothing. **Figure 13** shows two different types of hip protectors. There is also a style designed specifically for men. If you also have urinary incontinence, some styles allow for the use of pads.

Studies evaluating fractures in people using hip protectors have conflicting results; some show a benefit

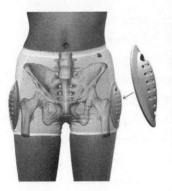

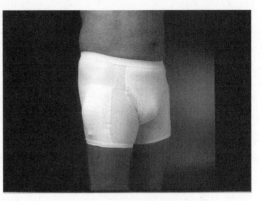

(a) A hip protector can provide cushioning over the hip bone.

(b) Hip protectors in washable underwear for men.

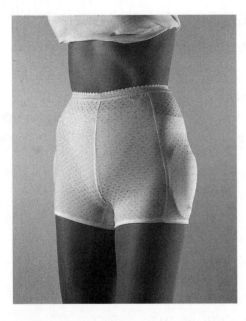

Figure 13   Styles of hip protectors. Courtesy of HIProtector® Fall Prevention Devices.

(c) Hip protectors in washable underwear for women.

and others do not. Although hip protectors can absorb up to 75% of the impact of a fall, one of the biggest problems with assessing their effectiveness in reducing fracture risk and probably the biggest barrier to their effectiveness is getting people to actually use them.

If your clinician suggests hip protectors, it's not something that will hurt you, so go ahead and use them. A number of medical–surgical supply companies carry hip protectors, and they are available on the Internet. It's important to measure yourself accurately so that the protectors don't slip around or dig into your hips. Because hip protectors can be expensive, shop around.

81. It's hard not to think about my bones being weak. How do I keep osteoporosis from interfering with my life?

Being told you have low bone mass or being diagnosed with osteoporosis can represent an opportunity for change. Rather than letting the news interfere with your life, think of it as an opportunity to make positive changes. Rather than feeling deprived or feeling old, let osteoporosis be a life-changing moment. Because osteoporosis is a "silent" disease, you probably did not know you had it. But some of the changes you make now can positively affect the rest of your life.

Once you are diagnosed, work to accomplish the following:

- *Stay positive.* A recent study of midlife men and women linked happiness with health. The happier you are, the healthier you are.
- *Get organized.* If you are on many medications and you are taking medication to prevent or treat osteoporosis, get yourself a pill-minder to make sure that you are taking your medication in the appropriate amount, on the correct day, and at the right time. Even if you only take a couple of medications, it's worth it to your peace of mind to get organized and

use a pill-minder so that by lunchtime, you don't
have to worry about whether you took your morning
dose of osteoporosis or blood pressure medication.

- *Resolve to get healthy.* Go to *www.mypyramid.gov*
and evaluate the diet that is right for you. Read as
much as you can about osteopenia and osteoporosis.
Make sure that you are getting regular check-ups
with clinicians for your overall health, including
dentists and vision care professionals. If you take
steroids, work with your clinician to reduce the
dosage or find other therapies that can reduce bone
loss (see Questions 87 and 88).

- *Develop goals directed at improving your bone health.*
Get enough calcium, vitamin D, and other substances necessary for good bone development. Make
lifestyle changes that directly affect bone such as
quitting smoking and reducing alcohol intake to a
moderate level (see Question 86). Take your medication faithfully.

- *Evaluate your environment for the potential for falls.*
Falls can happen to anyone. Taking action to review
the environment around you helps you and others
(see Question 79).

- *Above all, keep moving!* Develop an exercise routine
that you can stick with. Find ways of staying active
that you enjoy. Once you realize that osteoporosis
doesn't have to interfere with your life, you can
improve your bones while you improve your life!

82. In addition to osteoporosis, I have many health problems associated with midlife. I'm feeling very stressed. How can I keep from getting depressed?

It is not uncommon to feel stressed at midlife and into
your senior years. If you are in perimenopause, there is

a greater possibility of new depression during this time of your life. In fact, three times more women experience depression during perimenopause than at any other time prior to that. If you are a man at midlife, you may be having many of the same symptoms women experience during perimenopause and post-menopause, such as irritability, forgetfulness, and fatigue, or you may be experiencing the "midlife crisis" sometimes associated with disappointment after reviewing your life accomplishments.

Depression among older adults is common, too. In fact, depression and osteoporosis are physically and psychologically linked. Depression has been associated with low bone mass as well as increased risk of fracture. And if you fracture a bone, it is easy to become depressed from the lack of mobility, the social isolation, and the fear of falling or fracturing another bone (see Questions 2, 18, and 78).

Depression has been associated with low bone mass as well as increased risk of fracture.

Medications, medical conditions such as thyroid disorders, nutritional deficiencies, or stressful life events also can cause depression. According to the National Institute of Mental Health, any of the following symptoms that persist for longer than 2 weeks should be addressed by a mental health professional:

- A persistent sad, anxious, or empty mood
- Feeling hopeless or pessimistic
- Feeling guilty, worthless, or helpless
- Loss of interest or pleasure in hobbies or activities that you usually enjoy, including sex
- Prolonged tiredness, lack of energy
- Difficulty concentrating, remembering, and making decisions
- Difficulty falling or staying asleep, early morning awakening, or oversleeping

- Appetite or weight loss, or overeating and weight gain (stress eating)
- Thinking about death or about killing yourself
- Feeling restless or irritable
- Persistent physical symptoms that do not respond to treatment, such as headaches or stomach upset.

When you start to feel overly stressed, it's not too late to manage the stress to prevent the need for a mental health professional. There are plenty of stress management techniques that have been proven effective. The following are just a few of the ways to manage your stress:

- *Breathe.* Paced respiration can work well to keep you calm. Breathe in for the count of 4, hold your breath for 7 counts, and then breathe out for 8. Slow, rhythmic breathing can be done anytime.
- *Schedule time for yourself.* Make time to do some things that you especially enjoy. Read, watch a favorite television show or movie, take a walk, work on a hobby, or go to the gym.
- *Get a good night's sleep.* Lack of sleep feeds into the "stress–no-sleep" cycle, making stress worse.
- *Laugh loud and often.* Laughter releases endorphins in the brain, which will improve your mood.
- *Eat well.* A healthy diet can make you less irritable and more likely to resist stress and illness.
- *Exercise.* While it may sound like exercise is the answer to everything, it really can decrease your stress level. Exercising releases endorphins, substances that are associated with mood—and in a good way! A daily exercise routine has been suggested as a way to feel younger and look younger, great incentives for using exercise to reduce stress. Exercise is an inexpensive and effective prescription for feeling better about yourself, and a great way to help in the prevention and treatment of depression.

83. My mother has fractured vertebrae in her back several times. Is that common? How do I know if I fracture one of mine? How long will it take to heal?

Vertebral compression fractures (VCFs) account for half of all fractures related to osteoporosis. Although VCFs can cause extreme pain, they can also be "silent." In fact, two-thirds of spinal fractures do not cause pain. Regardless of pain, VCFs can lead to major changes in your mother's life:

- VCFs can cause loss of height. **Figure 14** shows an example of a spinal fracture, and Figure 6 (Question 18) shows the decrease in height as more vertebrae compress, shortening the spine.
- VCFs can bring about physiologic changes such as respiratory and gastrointestinal problems because the spine becomes compressed, which leads to pushing the body's internal organs together. Compression

Vertebral compression fracture (VCF)

A fracture of the body of a vertebra (spine bone) that collapses it and makes it thinner and weaker. Usually results from osteoporosis but can also result from complications of cancer or some injuries.

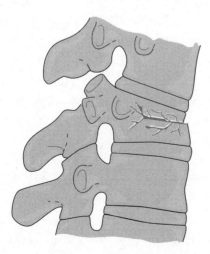

Figure 14   Vertebral compression fracture.

225

of the organs can result in shortness of breath, pain, reflux, incontinence, and indigestion.

- VCFs can cause a decreased quality of life. Your mother may not be able to do the things she has always done for herself. If she works outside the home, she may not be able to do her job. At home, her activities may be limited due to her inability to bend, reach, lift, and go up and down stairs. It may be difficult for her to bathe and dress herself. Unfortunately, the effects on her quality of life can continue even after the fracture heals.

- There is a 12-fold increase in the risk of fracturing another vertebra within 1 year. The anticipation of new fractures can be very scary. The loss of independence can cause mental health problems and a loss of self-esteem.

- VCFs can cause both acute and chronic back pain and sleeplessness.

- VCFs can cause depression and anxiety.

- Death rates are higher among those who have vertebral fractures. There is a 5% to 10% increase in all causes of death following a vertebral fracture. Shockingly, after 5 years following a spinal fracture, death rates go up by 20% beyond the rate expected for a person's age and sex. Clearly, it is important to prevent these fractures, detect and treat them if they occur, prevent future fractures, and attend to mental and physical health following a VCF.

- The financial burden for VCFs can also be high. Being out of work following a VCF or taking time out of work to care for a loved one with a VCF contributes to the high cost of fractures. There may be expenses for required care that are not covered by Medicare, Medicaid, or other insurance. In fact, it's estimated that only 83% of the costs related to osteoporosis is paid for by any type of insurance.

Because VCFs don't always cause pain, you may have one and not know it. Sometimes VCFs are suspected when your height is measured at your physical exam. A loss of height can be the first indication that you have had a VCF. Chest x-rays can also reveal fractures that have not been previously diagnosed. In a recent study, a staggering 75% of vertebral fractures noted on chest x-rays were among older adults who were not being treated for osteoporosis! Question 12 lists the risk factors for osteoporosis, so you can request BMD testing of your spine before you get a fracture.

Although VCFs can sometimes be seen on conventional x-rays, they are often missed. Multiple fractures can be missed, too. So further evaluation is usually needed, especially if you are experiencing back pain or have unexplained height loss and a conventional x-ray doesn't show a fracture. VCFs can be managed a couple of ways. If you have not been on medications for osteoporosis, your clinician will likely suggest treatment with a bisphosphonate. Fosamax reduces the incidence of vertebral fractures by 47% after 3 years and Actonel by 41% to 49%. Fosamax, Actonel, Boniva, and Reclast all increase BMD in the spine in women who have an existing vertebral fracture. So, while your current fracture is healing, you could be preventing future fractures by taking a bisphosphonate. In addition, you may be treated with Miacalcin NS or Fortical (calcitonin nasal spray) because the calcitonin spray helps slow bone breakdown and has pain-killing effects. However, calcitonin nasal spray is not usually a first-line treatment choice. Rather, it is used when bisphosphonate therapy cannot be tolerated or when Evista or Forteo cannot be used. Menopause hormone therapy is not the best option to start when

Because VCFs don't always cause pain, you may have one and not know it.

Living with Osteoporosis

you have a vertebral fracture because MHT is used for prevention, not treatment.

A few clinicians might prescribe a back brace, which needs to be correctly fitted. The brace, usually worn during the hours you are awake, prevents your spine from twisting or bending so that the fractures can heal more easily. It also serves as an instant reminder not to bend forward, twist, or flex the spine. **Figure 15** shows how a back brace is used to support the spine. A vertebral fracture can take from 6 to 8 weeks to heal. Although bed rest may be suggested initially, long stretches in bed are not recommended and do not heal fractures any faster. Your muscles can become very weak by staying in bed, which makes you less likely to tolerate activity and exercise. While back braces and bed rest were commonly used in the past, they are rarely recommended now because the risks of inactivity and the benefits of maintaining activity have been better recognized. In fact, bone loss that occurs while you are in bed is substantial. Vertebral bone loss in older adults on bed rest accelerates to 50 times the rate that occurs in young adults.

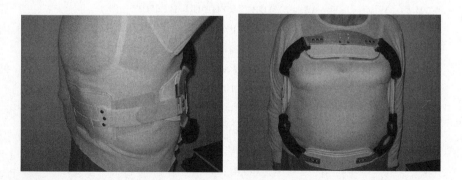

Figure 15   Example of a brace that provides support to the spine after a vertebral compression fracture.

Some clinicians will x-ray the spine again to determine progress. If you are no longer in pain, it doesn't necessarily mean that the fracture has healed completely, as many vertebral fractures do not cause pain in the first place. How you are feeling is the biggest guide for activity. You should slowly resume your normal activities as soon as possible, and avoid extended periods of inactivity. Your clinician likely will also want to monitor your bone density and measure your height regularly to screen for possible additional VCFs.

84. What is a "dowager's hump"? Can it be reversed?

The clinical term for "dowager's hump" is kyphosis. It's a bending forward of the top part of the spine causing a rounded hump appearance. Kyphosis is not the same as scoliosis, which is an "S" curve of the spine and is usually diagnosed in childhood or adolescence (**Figure 16**).

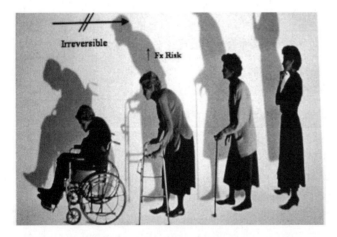

Figure 16 Osteoporosis can cause irreversible damage to the spine, leading to significant disability. Courtesy of the National Association of Nurse Practitioners in Women's Health (NPWH).

Progressive kyphosis eventually causes the abdomen to protrude. It came to be known by its colloquial name "dowager's hump" because it was traditionally noted in older women. The curving of the spine is caused by the collapse of the front of the vertebrae due to tiny fractures. (Figure 6 in Question 18 shows the progression of kyphosis.)

Once you reach a certain point in the curving of the spine, the kyphosis is not reversible. Figure 16 shows the progression from a spine unaffected by osteoporosis to the point at which the kyphosis resulting from osteoporosis cannot be reversed. After your fractures are healed, it is important to begin an exercise program to prevent kyphosis and to even reverse some of the curve before it reaches the point where it cannot be reversed. **Figure 17** shows exercises that can be done to stretch the muscles around the spine, increase flexibility, and reduce the likelihood of more fractures. These are great exercises to do even if you have never had a vertebral fracture, because they strengthen the muscles surrounding the spine.

85. What is kyphoplasty? Would it help my spinal fractures?

Spinal (or vertebral) fractures are a major concern for men and women with osteoporosis because they can lead to severe pain and disability (see Question 84). These fractures can also lead to kyphosis (see Figure 14 in Question 83). The spine deteriorates and curves due to fractures in individual vertebrae. Most osteoporotic vertebral fractures are traditionally treated with pain medications and a gradual return to normal activities. Although back braces to prevent twisting and support the spine were used in the past, they are infrequently

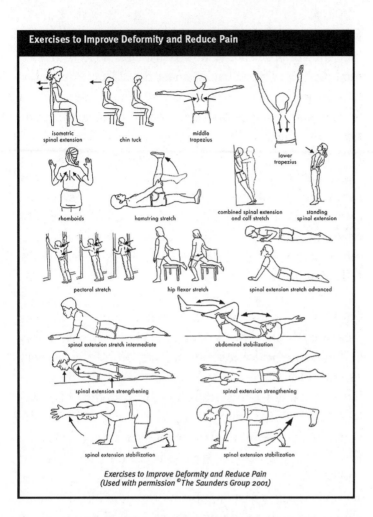

Exercises to Improve Deformity and Reduce Pain

Exercises to Improve Deformity and Reduce Pain
(Used with permission ©The Saunders Group 2001)

Figure 17   Exercises to prevent or improve deformity and reduce pain. Source: Duke University Medical Center's Bone and Metabolic Disease Clinic. Reprinted with permission. Gold DT, Lee LS, Tresolini CP, eds. *Working with Patients to Prevent, Treat, and Manage Osteoporosis: A Curriculum Guide for the Health Professions,* **3rd ed. Durham, NC: Center for the Study of Aging and Human Development, Duke University Medical Center; 2001.**

used today. Immobility associated with the brace or bed rest can increase the risk for blood clots, isolation, depression, and increased bone loss, and is usually not advised (see Question 83).

Kyphoplasty is a surgical procedure that helps to correct the collapse of the lumbar (lower back) and thoracic (mid to upper back) vertebrae. More important, this procedure can significantly reduce the pain of fractures and help individuals return to normal activities, sometimes within hours of surgery. Kyphoplasty is normally reserved for patients experiencing significant pain for at least 3 to 4 weeks, patients who may be in danger of developing bedsores from extended bed rest and immobility, and those who are not responding to conservative treatment. Kyphoplasty is more successful if performed within 2 to 3 months following the fracture.

For kyphoplasty, an incision is made in the spine under local anesthesia. The patient can be awake so that pain and neurological problems arising from the surgery can be immediately identified. An uninflated balloon-like instrument is inserted into the vertebra. The balloon is inflated, increasing the space within the vertebra. Sometimes this maneuver straightens the vertebra. Sometimes it doesn't. The balloon is removed and a special cement compound fills in the space, somewhat like a cast supporting the bone. Pain relief is almost immediate. Being able to resume normal daily activities can also be expected, thereby reducing the amount of disability caused by the vertebral fractures. Kyphoplasty is not a substitute for other treatments for osteoporosis, however. You may still need to take prescription medications, and you must take adequate calcium and vitamin D. You should also exercise regularly once your clinician has given you the go-ahead after surgery.

Kyphoplasty was originally based on the principles of **vertebroplasty,** which is a procedure usually performed by radiologists, who inject a cement-like substance into the fractured vertebrae using special x-ray techniques. This procedure does not require a surgical incision and does not use the balloon technique before cement is injected. Patients have said that they get immediate relief from the pain caused by the fractures.

Kyphoplasty is also used for patients with vertebral fractures resulting from metastases (that is, spread of disease from one part of the body to another) of cancers, which weaken bones, often in the spine. These fractures are extremely painful. The surgical procedure for fractures that result from metastases is often followed by radiofrequency waves to the affected areas of the spine.

86. Besides adding calcium and vitamin D, should I be changing anything in my diet? I heard that drinking alcohol could increase my risk of osteoporosis. Do I have to stop drinking entirely?

It's important to not only add calcium and vitamin D, but to make sure you are getting all of the necessary nutrients for bone growth, such as folate, phosphorus, magnesium, and protein. Evaluating your diet has become easier because the United States Department of Agriculture (USDA) has revamped its food pyramid to adjust for the many diseases and conditions affected by your diet and nutrition. Visit the new USDA Web site (*www.mypyramid.gov*) and find the food pyramid that is right for your age, gender, and physical activity level (see Questions 47–53). A recent study of men and women who ate a strict vegetarian raw food diet for up to 10 years showed that this type of diet is associated with lower bone density. Overall, the participants had an average BMI of 20, a known risk factor for osteoporosis, and they consumed no animal sources of calcium such as dairy products. However, because they spent more time in the sun than their nonvegetarian counterparts, they were not deficient in vitamin D. See Question 50.

Alcohol is an interesting paradox when it comes to osteoporosis. Although heavy alcohol consumption can bring about major social, financial, and health problems, mild to moderate consumption is associated with decreased rates of osteoporosis as well as decreased rates of heart attack, stroke, and diabetes. The Nurses' Health Study showed that women who drank moderate amounts of alcohol had higher bone mineral densities at the spine than their nondrinking counterparts. Heavy alcohol consumption, though, increases bone breakdown, meaning that you are more likely to have weaker bones. But since moderate consumption contributes in a positive way to bone formation, you can continue to drink moderately with a diagnosis of osteoporosis.

But what is moderate consumption? The latest dietary guidelines from the USDA recommend that alcohol intake be limited to one alcoholic beverage per day for women and two per day for men. One alcoholic beverage equals one 12-ounce beer, one 5-ounce glass of wine, or 1.5 ounces of hard liquor, such as vodka, rum, whiskey, etc. In general, red wine with a meal is commonplace in the Mediterranean countries, where heart disease is less frequent than in the United States. A glass of wine can be considered therapeutic, but you should remember that 5 ounces does not fill up the typical wine glass. Naturally, any amount of alcohol can impair your judgment and reflexes, so it's important not to drive, operate machinery, or engage in any activities that require skill and coordination if you have consumed alcohol.

Alcohol should be avoided by those who can't restrict the number of drinks they take, pregnant and breast-feeding women, women of childbearing age who may become pregnant, children and adolescents, those who are taking medications that are dangerous to combine with alcohol, and those with certain medical conditions.

None of the medications that are prescribed for osteo-porosis are dangerous to take with alcohol. However, if you are taking any of the bisphosphonates, you should always wait the required length of time (30 minutes to 2 hours) after taking the medication before eating or drinking anything.

87. Are there any medications that I should adjust or stop taking while I'm being treated for osteoporosis?

Presumably, you are taking prescription medications that are important to the treatment of your medical conditions. However, it's very important for you to be taking the smallest dosage that gives you the maximum benefit of any medication. Sometimes a medicine is prescribed by one clinician who is unaware of medication that you are taking that was prescribed by a different clinician. So, you need to be certain that all of your clinicians know about all of the medications you are taking. In addition, there are some over-the-counter medications such as nonsteroidal anti-inflammatory drugs (NSAIDs), like ibuprofen, aspirin, and naproxen, and antacids that can increase side effects or interfere with your new medications for osteoporosis.

In Question 15, there were certain medications mentioned that are good for bone health. There are other medications, however, that have a direct and negative impact on your bones (also see Question 15). If you are diagnosed with osteoporosis or placed on a medication to prevent further bone loss, you should have a detailed discussion with your clinician. Ask about possible interactions with any of your other medications and if any of the medications you are currently on can be eliminated or reduced in dosage. Decreasing the dosage can reduce some of the future effects of taking drugs that can negatively affect bone; however, you shouldn't sacrifice the drug's effectiveness by lowering the dose to the point at which it no longer serves its intended purpose.

If you are already taking estrogen, you may not take Evista. If your clinician wants you to opt for Evista, you must stop taking MHT. Forteo interacts with digoxin, increasing the possibility of digoxin toxicity, so your digoxin levels should be monitored carefully. The response to calcitonin nasal spray may be decreased if bisphosphonates (Actonel, Boniva, Fosamax, Reclast) are currently being taken or used immediately prior to the beginning of treatment with calcitonin nasal spray. However, calcitonin nasal spray may occasionally be prescribed for its pain-relieving effects following a VCF even if you are already taking a bisphosphonate.

With any of the bisphosphonates, you must never take any of your other medications at the same time as you are taking the bisphosphonate. Zantac (ranitidine), Prilosec (omeprazole), and other medications intended to reduce stomach acid should not be taken within 2 hours of a bisphosphonate. Because aspirin and other NSAIDs can increase stomach irritation and upset, they should be reduced in usage as much as possible if you are taking a bisphosphonate.

If you are immobilized from a fracture, you should stop taking estrogens or Evista because being sedentary can increase your risk of getting blood clots. Naturally, stopping any medications or restarting them should be done in consultation with your clinician.

88. I have been taking steroids for the treatment of my lupus. Is there any way that I can reduce the dosage so that the steroids do not further weaken my bones?

Systemic lupus erythematosis (SLE or lupus for short) and other inflammatory diseases, such as rheumatoid arthritis, inflammatory bowel diseases, and asthma, are often treated with steroids for long periods of time, but it does not take long for steroids to weaken bones. In fact, significant bone loss can occur with 5 mg or more per day in as little as 3 months. Courses of treatment for longer than 6 months give you a 50% chance of developing osteoporosis. So, in terms of your bones, it is critical to find ways to reduce your dosage of steroids or to begin medications such as a bisphosphonate and, if appropriate, estrogen therapies, that will help prevent further bone loss.

One of the alternative medications to steroids for rheumatoid arthritis and other autoimmune disorders is methotrexate, traditionally used for the treatment of cancers. Unfortunately, methotrexate can cause bone loss as well.

While you may not be able to lower your dose of steroids if your lupus is well controlled on your current dose, you likely can add medications that may make your bone loss less severe. But first make sure that you are doing everything that you can to make changes in your lifestyle that will improve your bone health. Get enough calcium and Vitamin D either through your diet or through supplementation. Exercise regularly. Nicotine can increase steroids' negative effect on bones, so it is particularly important that you stop smoking.

You and your clinician should discuss treatment with MHT (if you're a postmenopausal woman), bisphosphonates, calcitonin, and synthetic parathyroid hormone. Some clinicians recommend a discussion about medication options when their patients have been on steroids for as little as 3 months. Significant improvement in bone density can be made in just 1 year of therapy with Fosamax or Actonel in patients with glucocorticoid- (steroid-) induced osteoporosis (GIO), thereby reducing their risk of fracture.

dehydroepis-androsterone (DHEA)

A precursor to testosterone secreted by the adrenal glands and ovaries; in supplement form, made from steroid molecules extracted from wild yam, an herb.

For those who have lupus, a steroid called **dehydroepiandrosterone (DHEA)** may also offer some hope. DHEA is secreted in the human body by the adrenal glands, and in women the ovaries also make a small amount. In patients with lupus, DHEA levels are lower than normal. It is not clear from the research whether DHEA helps those with lupus, because it directly affects the mechanism that causes the disease, or if DHEA allows lower dosages of traditionally prescribed steroids, such as prednisone, to be effective.

By reducing prednisone dosages, the bone loss associated with it can be decreased.

The dietary supplement form of DHEA is made from steroid molecules extracted from wild yam, an herb that has been used for years to manufacture estrogen, progesterone, and testosterone. Because DHEA is a precursor of testosterone, sometimes high dosages of it cause male characteristic side effects such as facial hair and acne, although doses around 50 mg or less do not appear to cause these side effects. DHEA has been touted as an anti-aging miracle drug. Its claimed effects include increased energy and better sex drive. Although DHEA is available over the counter, you must discuss its pros and cons with your clinician before trying it. The dosage of DHEA being used in clinical trials is about 150 mg to 200 mg per day. A clinical trial looking at DHEA's effect on Crohn's disease is also being conducted.

Recent research studies showed that DHEA, when taken in conjunction with traditional lupus therapies, may improve bone density at the hip and spine, and may reduce lupus flares in women. Whether DHEA actually reduces flares of lupus, allows prednisone dosages to be reduced, or increases your BMD, DHEA may be worth discussing with your rheumatologist.

89. I recently overdid my weight-lifting. My knee is extremely swollen and painful. Am I more likely to have fractured a bone near my knee because I have osteoporosis?

Although you have an increased risk of fracture, it is more likely that you have strained the muscles and ligaments around your knee, causing it to be very swollen and painful when you walk on it. The fact that you over-did your weight-lifting is not surprising, particularly if you are newly diagnosed with osteoporosis. The tendency is to jump into an exercise program without regard for safety and overall conditioning. But it's important to maintain your enthusiasm while developing a sane and safe method of improving your bone health.

Weight-lifting can be very tricky, particularly if you are loading on the weights. If you are beginning a weight-lifting program at a fitness club, get instructions on how to use the machines that target certain muscle groups. You will want to make sure that you are using the correct technique before you add more weight. As we age, the knee joint deteriorates faster because it has had a lifetime of absorbing the greatest weight of any joints compared to its size. While hip joints are absorbing your weight as well, they are larger joints that can distribute your weight over your pelvic bones.

Knee joints wear out as a result of aging and osteoarthritis.

Knee joints wear out as a result of aging and osteoarthritis (see Question 96). Adding more weight to the stress already placed on your knees by your own weight may not be helpful and—worse—it can cause injury. If you are flexing and then extending your knee, with added weight, or extending and then flexing, your knee may not be able to tolerate this much stress at first. As a result, the cartilage, ligaments, or tendons around the knee can become inflamed. Cartilage is the rubbery connective tissue that is found in joints and the outer ear. Ligaments are tough bands that connect bones to each other, and tendons are also tough tissue bands that connect muscles to bones.

If your cartilage, ligaments, or tendons swell and become painful when you walk, you should first

"RICE" your knee: Rest, Ice, Compress, and Elevate. Stop doing exercises for at least several days, and most certainly do not resume the weight-lifting or exercise that caused the injury in the first place. Ice your knee periodically through the day while you're keeping it elevated. When you must walk on it, use a compression bandage such as an Ace wrap, winding it from below the knee upward to above the knee. If these measures do not relieve the knee pain, then you need to be evaluated by your clinician. If you cannot bear weight at all, you may need to use crutches, but sometimes crutches cause more problems than they're worth, particularly if they are not fitted properly to your height or you end up falling because you can't use them correctly. If the acute pain continues even when you're elevating your knee and not moving it, you should talk to your clinician about an x-ray. Although the bones around your knee are not likely to fracture as a result of weight-lifting, an x-ray may be helpful in diagnosing the degree of swelling and soft tissue injury your weight-lifting has caused, and may also be helpful in determining if there has been any shift in alignment of the knee due to the injury.

After your knee is fully healed, you should resume your exercise program. Take it slowly, begin with gentle stretching exercises, and gradually increase the number of repetitions and amount of weight that you use.

PART FIVE

Prevention and Going Forward

I'm worried that my daughter, who is 40, will get osteoporosis. How can she prevent this from happening to her?

What should I tell my family about osteoporosis? Will it curtail activities with them?

Osteoporosis seems to be featured in the news almost daily. What are some of the future treatments? Are there any new drugs that are being evaluated in clinical trials for the treatment of osteoporosis?

More...

90. I'm worried that my daughter, who is 40, will get osteoporosis. How can she prevent this from happening to her?

If you have already been diagnosed with osteoporosis, you are right to be concerned. Family history is certainly a risk factor for osteoporosis. But what you have learned from your own diagnosis can truly help your daughter.

Women beginning midlife should make themselves aware of all the risk factors for developing osteoporosis. First, at the age of 40, unless she is one of the 1% who experience premature menopause (natural and total cessation of menstrual periods before the age of 40), she is likely to still be making the necessary estrogen to protect her bones. She should continue to take adequate calcium and vitamin D for her age, which means 1000 to 1200 mg of elemental calcium and 400 IU of vitamin D per day. This may mean assessing her diet and supplementing it if she does not get enough calcium through dairy products and other foods (see Table 4 in Question 47). If she smokes, she should stop. If she drinks excessive alcohol, she should stop that, too. Equally important, she should develop an exercise routine that puts the necessary stress on her bones for them to continue to remodel appropriately. Making exercise a habit is critical to keeping bones strong through midlife and beyond (see Questions 43–45).

Making exercise a habit is critical to keeping bones strong through midlife and beyond.

If your daughter is 40 and also has asthma or one of the autoimmune disorders that require treatment with steroids, she needs to be aware that steroids can cause significant bone loss. She should consult her clinician about taking a medication that will help her maintain her bone density.

91. What about my granddaughter? She is only 16. Should I also worry about my grandson?

The importance of reaching peak bone mass cannot be overemphasized. Ninety percent of peak bone mass is reached by age 20 to 30. One of the periods of greatest bone growth occurs at the beginning of puberty (the other period is in infancy to toddlerhood). Boys must take in at least 1000 mg of calcium per day and girls must take in at least 850 mg of calcium per day in order to reach peak bone mass; however, the recommended intake of daily calcium is even higher: 1300 mg for both boys and girls aged 9 to 18 years. Recommended daily intake of vitamin D for boys and girls in this age group is 200 IU.

You should encourage your grandchildren—male and female—to do all the things that everyone at any age needs to do to have good bone health. Convincing teens to drink milk instead of soda sometimes feels like a losing battle. They should be encouraged to drink 2 to 3 glasses of skim or 1% milk per day, or get enough dairy products in their diet to get the calcium required for bone development and for them to reach their maximum height. Teens especially tend to drink soda or other non-nutritious beverages, and some drink as many as six cans of soda per day. Regrettably, they sometimes begin drinking alcoholic beverages or start smoking at an early age. These poor health habits can harm their bone development.

Although teens often get good sources of dietary calcium by eating cheese on pizza or cheeseburgers, low-fat dairy products should be encouraged as well, such as yogurt, puddings, and low-fat cheese. Because of the high sugar and fat content of many popular foods, adolescents need to get the necessary calcium for bones without increasing their risk of obesity. They can also get calcium from fortified orange juice, cereals, and even Calci-Fresh chewing gum, which contains calcium. Vitamin D is available in fortified dairy and cereal products. An added incentive for your granddaughter is that diets higher in calcium and vitamin D have recently been shown to help prevent premenstrual syndrome (PMS).

Urging teens and helping them to quit smoking is another challenge. Smoking cessation programs are often not successful, even in the face of gory lung cancer photos. But studies in teens have shown they are more responsive to messages about ugly stained teeth and bad breath as a result of smoking than negative health consequences. Pictures of osteoporotic bones are not likely to make teens quit smoking either, especially if they think this couldn't happen to them until they're much older. But still, making an effort to focus on the future negative impact on their appearance, particularly the hunched back, may have a positive result.

Many teens have cars now, so unless they are on sports teams at school, they are less likely to be getting a significant amount of exercise. They should be reminded of the benefits of walking to a friend's house, and few teens have to be encouraged to go to the mall to walk around. Thirty to sixty minutes of moderate exercise per day should be their goal. Exercise routines developed in adolescence are more likely to be carried into adulthood.

The sport of weight-lifting has gained increasing popularity among young adults. Weight-lifting is different from strength training. Strength training uses free weights, one's own body weight, machines, or elastic bands to exert resistance on muscles. While strength training does increase strength and puts appropriate stress on bones, it does so without increasing muscle mass in children and adolescents who have not reached puberty. Strength training should be encouraged in all age groups and is appropriate for children and adolescents as long as they can follow directions and receive adequate adult supervision. Improving strength will depend on the intensity, frequency, duration, and type of strength training. Weight-lifting, the competitive sport of lifting weights with specified technique and movements, should not be started before the completion of puberty. Adolescents should be advised against using anabolic steroid supplements to put on muscle mass, as they actually cause bone to break down and weaken.

Strength training should be encouraged in all age groups and is appropriate for children and adolescents as long as they can follow directions and receive adequate adult supervision.

There are certain children and adolescents who are at special risk for not reaching their peak bone mass and for developing osteoporosis. Diseases and conditions that put them at risk include anorexia nervosa and bulimia, gastrointestinal diseases that affect their intestinal absorption such as gluten or lactose intolerance, chronic kidney and liver diseases, amenorrhea (no menstrual periods), autoimmune disorders that require treatment with steroids, and endometriosis that is treated with GnRH analogs (see Question 92). These young people should be monitored carefully for bone development and bone mass.

A study done recently showed that if teens get the recommended amount of calcium, their high-protein, high-salt, and high-phosphorus diets don't interfere with bone development. If, however, their soda intake substitutes for other sources of calcium, they are not likely to get the calcium they need.

Prevention and Going Forward

Delia's comment:

I wasn't prepared to hear that my teenage daughter might have osteoporosis. When we went to see an orthopedic specialist about her stress fractures, he asked if she had been exercising excessively. She had complained of severe back pain ever since she started running but he wasn't convinced at first that the amount of her running added up to stress fractures, which were diagnosed on MRI. Then he asked about any eating disorders, her periods, and the amount of calcium and vitamin D she was getting. Since she has never had an eating disorder or lost her periods from overexercising and she has a healthy diet, the doctor went on to ask about our family history. My mother has osteoporosis and I also have bone loss. We are both on treatment, she with Actonel, and I with Fosamax. Both of us take calcium and vitamin D supplements. Because of her family history and the stress fractures, my daughter was sent for bone mineral density testing of her spine and hips, which showed she did have osteopenia. She is being treated with extra calcium and 800 IU of vitamin D. She is also going for intensive physical therapy and strength training so that she will eventually be able to tolerate high impact sports again. My daughter has always been a good milk drinker, so I've never been concerned that she wasn't getting enough calcium and vitamin D, but now we can remind each other about calcium and exercise!

92. My daughter's friend is only 26 and has recently been diagnosed with osteoporosis as a result of being treated for endometriosis. Is osteoporosis reversible at her age?

Endometriosis is a condition usually diagnosed in teenage girls and young women but can still affect older menstruating women. It is characterized by severe pain and is caused by menstrual tissue that has migrated from the inside of the uterus to the outside of the uterus and attached to pelvic and abdominal organs, such as the ovaries, bladder, and intestines. Endometriosis can be treated by laparoscopic surgery, during which the migrated tissue is removed.

Endometriosis is often treated with birth control pills. And severe forms of endometriosis are sometimes treated with gonadotropin-releasing hormone (GnRH) analogs (e.g., Lupron [leuprolide]), which suppress menstrual cycles, effectively placing the woman in menopause. No matter what your age is, your bones will be affected if you are taking GnRH analogs for an extended period. It is now more commonly recommended that Lupron treatment be limited to 3 to 6 months at a time. If a young woman has been among those treated for years at a time, it is important for her bone density to be checked and appropriate treatment started.

Yes, at this age, osteoporosis can be reversed if she is treated with the necessary calcium, vitamin D, and, sometimes, an osteoporosis medication on the recommendation of a specialist. Once Lupron has been stopped, estrogen can once again be secreted normally or ingested through birth control pills, patches, or rings. The body's estrogen or that from prescribed estrogen will once again provide one of the necessary building blocks for bone. Once her bone density has increased and stabilized, any medications can usually be stopped unless another course of Lupron is anticipated. If birth control is not being used to continue treatment for endometriosis, a very reliable method of birth control must be used while taking any medication for osteoporosis.

Janelle's comment:

In the December that I was 22, I was diagnosed with osteoporosis. It was not exactly what I had expected for Christmas that year, and it brought with it some changes in my lifestyle. The real story begins some 10 years earlier, when I got my period for the first time. I went through about 20 pads the first day and had cramps so painful I could barely walk. The next time was no better, and I could add fainting to my list of symptoms. I soon learned that I had advanced endometriosis along with a cyst on one of my fallopian tubes. The surgeon removed the cyst and removed what he could of the endometriosis. Then he explained that I would have to go on a very strong medicine for 6 months to kill the rest of the endometriosis. I could only stay on this medicine, Lupron, for 6 months because it could reduce my bone density if used for longer. After the 6 months, I would go on other medications.

A day or two after my first Lupron injection I woke up crying and could not stop. I was so sad and I did not know why. I cried for days and finally learned that it was my body's reaction to the hormone adjustments caused by the Lupron. Well, I guess I adjusted, because the crying stopped and I did feel better. The Lupron had some other effects as well, namely that I would not have my period while on it. I also experienced hot flashes and night sweats. After the 6 months, I stopped the Lupron and went on a plan of "continuous birth control pills" for about 4 years.

I had surgery again when I was 17 to remove the endometriosis that had grown back during the ineffective continuous birth control pill (BCP) treatment. After this surgery the doctor explained that more research had been done on Lupron since the last time I used it, and there was evidence that one could stay on it for longer periods of time.

Since it had worked so well for me, and since the BCPs had worked so poorly, he suggested that I would be a good candidate to go on Lupron for a longer period of time.

In order to reduce the side effects of Lupron and allow me to stay on it for even longer, I began taking a combination of estrogen and progesterone normally prescribed for women in menopause. After 2 years on Lupron and the "add-back" hormone treatments, I had a bone density scan. The results were fine and I could stay on the treatment. I had another scan a year later and it was still OK, the doctor said. Sometime around the fourth year of the treatment, I was about to begin graduate school and switched to a different gynecologist. Since the treatment had been working so well, my new doctor suggested I stay on it at least for another year while I studied abroad.

I went home to see my parents for Christmas that year and while I was there, I had another bone density scan. Christmas was lovely, but the night before I was supposed to leave to go back to school, my doctor called to tell me that I had osteoporosis. I was shocked. I had all those bone scans along the way that were fine and the treatment seemed to be working so well—I had had no period pain for years. He explained that I would have to go off the Lupron immediately and begin taking Fosamax. I would also need to get calcium and vitamin D supplements and eat food to get at least 1500 mg of calcium a day.

When I got back to school, I went to the grocery store. Here in the United States, foods are required to list the amount of calcium they contain. The same is not true outside this country. Some products list it and others don't, so I did my best guessing job and loaded up my basket with yogurt, milk, cheese, and pudding. As time went on, I got more creative with my calcium: instant potatoes made with milk, dry soups made with milk, hot chocolate, and such. The Lupron took a while to wear off, as I had been on it for so long, and I did not get my period again for several months.

The following Christmas, 1 year after having been originally diagnosed, I went in for another bone test. The results were very promising: I had regained over 10% of my bone mass. All of those yogurts and string cheeses had paid off. While I am still taking Fosamax (and single handedly keeping yogurt companies in business), my bones are on their way to recovery. In about 2 more years, my doctor estimates that I should have complete recovery of my bone density.

93. I thought I heard that it is better to live in a warmer climate to prevent osteoporosis. Is that true?

Warm weather would not prevent osteoporosis. There would be no mechanism for it to do that. In fact, the rates of hip fractures are higher among southern states in the United States, probably due to the higher percentage of older individuals living in those areas. However, there are some advantages to warmer climates when it comes to preventing and treating osteoporosis.

For example, a warmer climate usually means being outside more. Although you are likely to get more exposure to sunshine (Question 51), the amount of sun exposure needed to provide enough vitamin D is too variable to count on for your daily dose of vitamin D. Additionally, most clinicians recommend regular use of sun block. So, use sun block regularly and take a vitamin D supplement daily.

Warmer climates make it easier for you to exercise out-doors. You are much more likely to walk outside when the weather is warmer year-round. This would give you incentive to get at least 30 minutes of exercise daily. Exercise, as you know by now, is critical to keep-ing your bones strong. Sometimes cold weather can make chronic conditions, such as arthritis, feel worse. Increased pain may prevent you from getting your necessary exercise (see Question 96).

If you don't have snow and ice to worry about, you're much less likely to fall, at least outside during the winter. That's certainly a big relief for people who have watched their every step in slippery conditions!

94. I'm 60 years old. Is it really worth it to start exercising now? Will exercise at my age help prevent osteoporosis?

Absolutely! Exercising will help you no matter how old you are. Although exercise has been encouraged for many years as part of a healthy lifestyle, we are just beginning to quantify its positive effects on heart dis-ease, obesity, diabetes, menopausal symptoms, and of course osteoporosis. It is never too late to incorporate regular exercise into your lifestyle. It's easy for us to say that we're too old to begin exercising at our age, but that is not true.

If you don't already have osteoporosis or osteopenia, exercise is still important even though exercise alone doesn't prevent bone loss. When you are well past the first 4 to 8 years after menopause, during which the greatest amount of bone loss occurs, and if you don't have osteoporosis, you are less likely to develop osteoporosis. If you are only a few years into post-menopause, you may still lose enough bone to be diagnosed with osteoporosis later. Regardless of how many years you are past menopause, get moving! And if you're a man, you should get moving, too. Men don't have to worry about estrogen loss with menopause, but they are still growing older, and that means bone loss.

Because your fracture risk is not only dependent on bone mineral density but also on bone quality, exercising regularly can strengthen your bones and possibly increase both density and quality. Exercise improves balance and coordination, reducing your risk of falling and also of fracture. It's always worthwhile to begin an exercise program after making sure that you have had a recent physical exam to rule out any conditions or abnormalities that would prevent you from engaging in regular exercise. You should start a program of exercise very slowly to build stamina and strength over time (see Question 45).

95. What's the likelihood that I will die from osteoporosis?

Osteoporosis itself will not be the direct cause of your death, but it can certainly contribute to an earlier-than-expected death. Your risk of dying following a hip fracture is up to 4 times more likely than peers in your age group who have not fractured a hip. In fact, 65,000 women die every year following a hip fracture. Women outnumber men when it comes to hip fractures, but men are more likely to die as a result of a hip fracture. In addition, if you do sustain a fracture, which is the most devastating result of osteoporosis, your quality of life can be markedly decreased. Many people who fracture a hip enter a nursing home in order to receive continuing care, and never regain their independence. Many end up dying in the nursing home.

With life expectancy increasing, the federal government is making recommendations in an effort to help you live out your years in a more healthful manner. By 2010, it is expected that 12 million men and women over the age of 50 will have osteoporosis, and a remarkable 40 million will have osteopenia. Preserving your bone health can help prevent osteoporosis and the fractures that can cause early death. Healthy People 2010, an initiative from the Department of Health and Human Services, challenges Americans to improve their health by engaging in activities that promote their overall well-being. Some of the challenges relate directly to bone health, such as avoiding tobacco and alcohol, as well as increasing activity and eating a healthy diet. For example, one of the goals of Healthy People 2010 is to reduce the percentage of adult Americans who smoke by half (from 24% to 12%). Another goal is to double the percentage of adults who exercise 30 minutes daily from 15% to 30%.

96. I have joint pain. Is that related to my osteoporosis? What can I do for the joint pain? Exercise seems to make the joint pain worse.

Joint pain usually results from wear and tear on the cartilage, causing osteoarthritis to develop. This type of arthritis causes inflammation and pain in the joints. The cartilage usually provides a buffer between the bones in your joints. When it is injured from years of weight bearing and activity, you can develop joint pain and osteoarthritis. While you might think that exercising would cause more discomfort, injure the joint, and increase joint degeneration, it does not. It is more damaging to your health to carry around extra weight and to develop weak muscles and bones. In a recent small study, regular moderate exercise (aerobic and weight-bearing activities for 1 hour, 3 times per week) was associated with improved physical activity and knee joint function as well as improved strength of knee cartilage.

It's important to exercise even when you have joint pain, although extra pain in the joints more than 2 hours after exercise may indicate that you have overexercised.

It's important to continue to exercise even when you have joint pain, although extra pain in the joints more than 2 hours after exercise may indicate that you have overexercised. Exercise will increase your strength, balance, flexibility, and cardiovascular fitness. Strengthening your muscles around your joints will help reduce the stress on them. For example, doing exercises that build thigh muscles can help reduce knee pain and improve its ability to support your weight. Some of the exercises featured in Appendix A can be done while seated to strengthen your thigh muscles.

Like your knees, your back is also susceptible to osteoarthritis. Chronic low back pain can result from the deterioration of the joints in your spine. Research evidence shows that both acute (lasting less than 6 weeks) and chronic low back pain do respond to exercise, especially stretching and strengthening exercises.

If you experience pain in the joints immediately following exercise, use an ice pack wrapped in a towel for about 20 minutes. If the pain persists, avoid the exercise and specific activities that cause pain, and continue to use ice several times a day for a few days. After a few days of using ice packs, warm therapies such as hot packs and whirlpool baths may ease joint pain better. Prolonged rest used to be prescribed for muscle or bone pain, but that is not the case now. Clinicians and scientists now recognize that immobility does more harm than good, so it's important to keep moving.

In one recent study of postmenopausal women, those taking Fosamax (alendronate) for osteoporosis had less knee pain and fewer abnormalities of their knee joints related to osteoarthritis. Further study is needed to determine if bisphosphonates like Fosamax have positive and preventive effects on osteoarthritis and joint pain.

Marjory's comment:

I think my osteoarthritis started in my knees about 20 years ago when I used to work as a nurse. Although I can't blame everything on walking daily on the hospital's cement floors, I'm sure it probably contributed to my knee problems. At the same time, I was taking exercise classes at a local Y where the floors were also cement but we wore improper shoes—you know, the kind of canvas sneakers that don't give you any support. Even back then, though, I realized the importance of exercise and have always exercised no matter how much my joints were bothering me. I discovered water aerobics about 10 years ago and went to the pool twice a week. I also did exercises at home. But once the physical aspects of patient care became too difficult with my arthritis, I retired. In addition to taking prescription anti-inflammatory medication for pain, I also had my knees injected with cortisone and Synvisc. But in spite of these therapies, 2 years ago I had both knees replaced because I had no cartilage left in the joints. It felt like bone was rubbing against bone. Now, there's no pain in my knees, although I continue to have pain in my shoulders, hips, ankles, and elbows. Less than a year ago, I was also diagnosed with rheumatoid arthritis. Now I exercise four times a week in a warm water pool with a water aerobics class. I also do Pilates classes in the water, on a big plastic ball, and in a chair. I lift weights for upperbody strength, and I also lift weights with my ankles to strengthen my legs. Then I burn about 65 calories walking on the treadmill, and now I wear good footwear meant for exercising. On my day off from exercising, I volunteer at the local library where I do lots of bending and stretching and even climbing on ladders! I can probably bend, stretch, and climb better because I do exercise regularly. Since I had gastrointestinal bleeding last fall, probably as a result of taking anti-inflammatory pain medications without stomach medication, I don't take much for pain any longer. No matter what, I keep up with my exercise. Even though I have painful joints, exercising allows me to sleep.

97. What should I tell my family about osteoporosis? Will it curtail activities with them?

If you have been diagnosed with osteoporosis, you should definitely discuss the diagnosis with your partner. First, your partner should know if you are on any new medications so he or she can help support you in following the new regimen and watch for reactions. Second, you and your partner should discuss how your lives might be affected by osteoporosis.

New medications can present some challenges to your schedule and that of your partner. If you are taking one of the bisphosphonates, you will need to establish the appropriate timing for taking your new medication. Sometimes, it's helpful for a partner or spouse to know that you must take the medication on first rising, to remain upright after taking it, and to avoid all other food, drink, and medication for at least 30 minutes to 2 hours. If your children are still living at home, they may help remind you as well. Sometimes, until the routine of taking certain medications gets ingrained in us, we may forget and take all of our medications at one time, which can cause serious side effects or reactions or make the medication less effective.

If your clinician has restricted your activity, discuss these restrictions with your partner or spouse and children. It is unlikely that you will be restricted from specific activities unless they are new to you (e.g., ice skating, skiing, skydiving). If you don't exercise regularly, this is a good time to discuss a new routine of exercising with your partner and children. Osteoporosis should not limit your activities or your thinking. Consider taking a class together for dancing, yoga, or tai chi.

A diagnosis such as osteoporosis also gives you the opportunity to discuss other lifestyle changes that may be helpful to your own, your partner's and your children's bone health and general health. Plan meals that will enhance your calcium and vitamin D intake. Quit smoking together. Make a pact with your partner to restrict alcohol to one glass of wine with dinner, or one cocktail or beer per day.

In addition to routines around exercise and medications, this might be a good time to assess your environment for the risks associated with falling. Take a good look at the inside and outside of your house or living space. Even if you think you're not old enough to be at risk for falling, everyone can benefit from removing clutter and putting up railings and good lighting (see Table 18 in Question 79).

98. My friends are all very health-conscious, and I believe they will think it's my fault that I have osteoporosis. My friends enjoy adventures like hiking, rock-climbing, and cross-country skiing. Must I decline their invitations to go with them?

Learning that you have osteopenia or being diagnosed with osteoporosis does represent an opportunity to help yourself and educate others.

Like other medical conditions and diagnoses, there are many factors that can put you at risk for osteoporosis. Many of them are factors that you cannot control. Your friends should not blame you for having osteoporosis, nor should you blame yourself. Blame serves no useful purpose. Learning that you have osteopenia or being diagnosed with osteoporosis does represent an opportunity to help yourself and educate others.

People who take adequate calcium and vitamin D and exercise regularly still get osteoporosis. So even though your friends are health conscious, it's possible for any of them to have or develop osteoporosis, too. Depending on your comfort level with discussing personal health information, it may be helpful to discuss your diagnosis with your friends. You might start the conversation with, "I just had one of those tests that measures bone density. Have any of you had one yet?" You will probably be surprised with their answers: "My doctor says I don't need one yet, but he also said I should increase my calcium," or "My mother just started using a nasal spray for a fracture in her back that happened because she has osteoporosis," or "No. How was the test? Was it painful?"

You can let your friends know what your clinician said, for example, about lifestyle changes; medications, foods, and supplements to take; and the types of exercise that are appropriate. Then, if your adventurous friends invite you to an activity that you cannot engage in, you are able to say, "Remember when I got the diagnosis of osteoporosis? I'm not able to go skiing [for example], but I could join you for dinner afterward." Or better yet, suggest and organize activities that you know will not prevent your participation. For example, you could organize a group to join a walk-a-thon, which would not only benefit each of you in terms of exercise and social interaction, but would also benefit worthy charities.

An open discussion of your diagnosis might even prompt your friends to ask their own clinicians about being tested or about making some changes in their own lifestyles. It's a blessing to have friends who want to be active, so don't let osteoporosis interfere with sharing many new adventures with your friends.

99. Osteoporosis seems to be featured in the news almost daily. What are some of the future treatments? Are there any new drugs that are being evaluated in clinical trials for the treatment of osteoporosis?

Osteoporosis and bone health are receiving much more notice in the news. Studies of the bones of certain animal species are spurring newer studies to see if those results are applicable to humans. There are several examples. The majority of growth in the bones of lambs takes place during the night when the lambs are sleeping, presumably when there is less pressure on their bones. This might account for children's complaints of growing pains at night. Purring is believed to be one of the factors responsible for the fast healing experienced by cats. Sound treatment in the same sound range as a cat's purr is being investigated to improve bone growth in older adults.

The role of fluoride in building good bone has been evaluated in large scale studies, but with discouraging results. Sodium fluoride as a supplement in baby vitamins and in drinking water has been around for years, and is responsible for helping to prevent tooth cavities. It is not clear from the studies if fluoridated drinking water affects bone mineral density. In one study of postmenopausal women in the Midwest, hip and vertebral fractures were decreased but wrist fractures were increased. A certain amount of fluoride is important for strong bone development, but excessive amounts are believed to cause the bones to become brittle because fluoride increases bone density but produces bone of very poor quality. Fluoride supplements are not currently recommended for the treatment of osteoporosis.

Livial (tibolone) is a synthetic steroid compound that has estrogen-, testosterone-, and progestin-like activity but does not contain any of these hormones. Although prescribed in 70 other countries, the FDA has not approved it, so it is not available in the United States. Studies have shown that tibolone used by postmenopausal women can increase bone mineral density and decrease bone turnover. Tibolone also significantly reduces hot flashes in postmenopausal women and is being studied as a medication to treat sexual dysfunction because of its androgenic effects. In a study of older women, tibolone was shown to reduce fracture risk at rates comparable to those of bisphosphonates, raloxifene, and hormone therapy. In this same study, tibolone was also shown to reduce the risk of invasive breast cancer and colon cancer. Since many women are seeking an alternative to estrogen therapy, it was hoped that tibolone would be approved in the United States; however, the FDA voted against its approval. Like all drugs, tibolone has some risk—it has been shown to increase the risk for stroke.

Osteoprotegerin is a substance known to decrease bone breakdown by preventing osteoclast formation (the cells that break down bone). Some research shows that human estrogen (17-β estradiol) and dietary phytoestrogens (see Question 54) can increase levels of osteoprotegerin and therefore reduce bone breakdown. Further research is needed before increased phytoestrogen intake can be recommended. A synthetic isoflavone (one of the phytoestrogens) called ipriflavone is still being studied for its long-term effects, because while there is evidence that it increases bone density, other evidence shows that ipriflavone may cause abnormally low white blood cell counts.

AMG-162, now known as denosumab, recently completed phase III clinical trials and was reviewed in October of 2009 by the FDA for approval for postmenopausal osteoporosis treatment and for treatment of bone loss from hormonal ablation therapy for breast or prostate cancer. It is also being investigated for treatment of rheumatoid arthritis, bone metastases, and multiple myeloma. Denosumab is a monoclonal antibody that acts like osteoprotegerin and interferes with the effects of a protein (RANK ligand). The RANK ligand protein causes bone loss. By interfering with this protein, denosumab inhibits the cells that cause bone breakdown (osteoclasts) and thus allows greater bone formation. Denosumab is administered by injection into the fat tissue (subcutaneous tissue) like Forteo. Unlike Forteo, which is given daily over a period of several months and only to those who do not respond to first-line treatment, denosumab is a first-line treatment agent and only needs to be given once every 6 months. The medication showed a significant increase in bone density and was well tolerated in phase III clinical trials. It also compared favorably with alendronate for both efficacy (bone density, serum markers, and urinary markers) and side effects in research studies. The FDA requested additional information for denosumab, which has a proposed trade name of Prolia. This information will be provided by the pharmaceutical manufacturer (Amgen) and approval is anticipated in 2010. Prolia will provide an important alternative for osteoporosis treatment. The subcutaneous injection is almost painless and can be self-administered at home or given at your clinician's office. It may be easier to remember than a daily or monthly pill and does not need the complex regimen required for taking oral bisphosphonates.

Another human monoclonal antibody, AMG 785, has shown promise in increasing the rate of bone formation. This works by interfering with the usual processes that limit bone formation in the body. A phase II clinical trial is expected for further evaluation of this possible therapy.

Preos, another parathyroid hormone in development, is being investigated for its effects on building bone. It is being evaluated for use in a cyclic dose (once-a-week injection after 3 months of daily injections) and also for its effects when used in combination with other therapies such as bisphosphonates.

Pamidronate, another bisphosphonate, is currently used in the treatment of high calcium levels and bone problems associated with some cancers. It is being studied as a treatment for osteoporosis, particularly in the population undergoing dialysis. Men and women who have chronic kidney disease have significant problems with calcium regulation and bone loss. Pamidronate has been effective in increasing bone density in healthy postmenopausal women when it was administered every 3 months, and studies have shown that a small protective effect on bone density persists after the medication is stopped. Pamidronate is usually given intravenously.

Although not yet approved by the FDA for use in the United States, Strontium ranelate, (Protelos, developed by Servier), a radionuclide, has been studied in Europe and Australia. Research shows that oral strontium ranelate not only increases BMD but also decreases both vertebral and nonverterbral fractures. This new medication represents an alternative for postmenopausal women who cannot tolerate other treatments for osteoporosis. It works by both increasing bone formation (increasing osteoblast activity) and reducing bone resorption (decreasing osteoclast activity). Strontium ranelate is taken orally and is already approved for use in several other countries, including Europe. Other forms of strontium—strontium malonate, strontium carbonate, and strontium citrate—are also being studied for use.

Arzoxifene, a new SERM or estrogen agonist/antagonist being developed by Eli Lilly and Co., completed phase III clinical trials in 2009 with promising results. In this study (called "FOUNDATION") women received 20 mg of the medication each day, plus calcium 500 mg. After 2 years, results indicated that bone mineral density had a statistically significant increase of 2.9% at the spine and 2.2% at the hip over placebo. In another study (called "NEXT"), arzoxifene was compared to Evista (another Lilly product) and demonstrated higher increases in BMD in the hip, spine, and femoral neck area. Arzoxifene was initially developed as a possible breast cancer medication, but tamoxifene proved better at reducing recurrence and women on tamoxifene were disease free longer. An ongoing study (called "GENERATIONS"), is further evaluating the effects of arzoxidene on bone, breast tissue, heart disease, and the uterus. Results from GENERATIONS are expected late in 2009.

Another new possibility is a combination of medications manufactured in one tablet. One such combination currently under investigation combines estrogen and a new estrogen agonist/antagonist. While taking Evista (raloxifene) and estrogen together is contraindicated because the medications compete for the same receptor sites, new estrogen agonists/antagonists that do not carry this contraindication are under investigation. A new estrogen agonist/antagonist that is more selective is being evaluated for combination with estrogen (in the same pill) for the treatment of postmenopausal osteoporosis in women who are also experiencing menopausal symptoms.

One of the new, more selective estrogen agonist/antagonists has shown success in reducing fractures. Bazedoxifene (BZA) is being evaluated by the FDA for osteoporosis prevention and treatment. Research has shown beneficial reductions in fractures (40% fewer fractures at the spine and 46% fewer on nonspine bones) without increasing risks for breast or endometrial cancers. BZA has also been studied in combination with conjugated equine estrogens as a tissue-selective estrogen complex (TSEC). So far results look promising, as this combination reduces symptoms associated with menopause, effectively preserves and strengthens bone, and does not increase risks for breast or endometrial cancer. This combination has also been shown to improve vaginal symptoms as well as sexual function and enjoyment in postmenopausal women.

Lasofoxifene is another new EAA that has been shown to slow bone turnover and increase bone density. Lasofoxifene reduced fractures in the spine and other areas and did not increase the risk for stroke, heart disease, or endometrial cancer. It somewhat increased the risk for blood clots, however it also reduced the risk for breast cancer. While still under investigation, this agent may become available in the future for osteoporosis management.

Therapies aimed at interrupting the bone resorption process in new ways are also being developed. One such compound, an integrin antagonist, currently called L-000845704, works by interfering with how osteoclasts attach to the bone surface. When osteoclasts cannot effectively attach to bone, the process of resorption is slowed. This compound increased bone density and decreased bone markers in a study done with postmenopausal women. Another compound, called odanacatib, is a selective inhibitor of cathepsin K. Cathepsin K is produced by osteoclasts to break down bone. Odanacatib inhibits bone resorption by interfering with the action of cathepsin K.

Other developments in osteoporosis treatment have to do with new ways to give established medications. For example, an oral form of salmon calcitonin is being evaluated. Salmon calcitonin is already available in nasal spray and injectable forms. Additionally, a transdermal form of human parathyroid hormone (PTH 1-34, Forteo) has shown some promise in increasing bone density. PTH 1-34 is also being evaluated for administration by mouth, nasal spray, and inhalation.

It's also important to keep your eyes and ears open for health care developments that are not specifically related to osteoporosis. For example, the statin drugs long used as treatment for high cholesterol levels may still prove to increase bone density, an indirect and positive result of drugs intended to lower unhealthy levels of cholesterol. And there is news in the nutrition world almost daily. For example, a recent study on rats showed less bone loss in the rats fed a particular substance (GPCS) found in white onions. Also, people who have gluten intolerance (celiac disease) have high rates of osteoporosis because they cannot effectively absorb calcium and vitamin D through their intestines. The gluten intolerance causes diarrhea, making it difficult for nutrients to be absorbed from the intestines because foods move through too quickly. When placed on gluten-free diets, the diarrhea stops and normal amounts of calcium and vitamin D can be absorbed, thereby improving bone density.

There is more osteoporosis news for men, too, particularly for those over the age of 65 who are trying to lose weight. Men in this age range should be wary about weight loss because it is associated with bone loss in the hip. Their clinicians should be monitoring both weight loss and bone loss. Although further study is needed, the potential for bone loss and the increased risk of fracture should be a topic of discussion between you and your clinician when weight loss is being recommended.

Bones will still require, at the very least, calcium, vitamin D, and exercise to stay strong.

It is quite common for an aging spine to look like the one featured in **Figure 18**, but it's more difficult to imagine that this spine can eventually look like the one in **Figure 19**. There is no instant cure for a disease that can cause such a deformity. Even future treatments will not be a cure. Bones will still require, at the very least, calcium, vitamin D, and exercise to

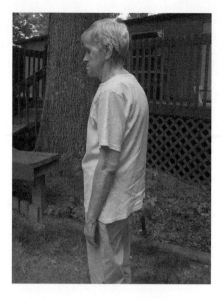

Figure 18 Many women have this degree of kyphosis. It can progress to a severe form in which organs are compressed and disability can be significant, as shown in Figure 19. Photo courtesy of Janet Wise.

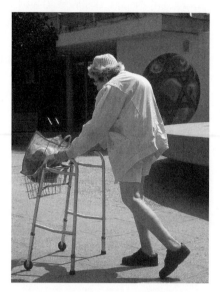

Figure 19 Woman with severe kyphosis (also known as "dowager's hump"). © Bill Aron/PhotoEdit, Inc.

stay strong. As addressed in Part 3, there are lifestyle changes and various therapies that can improve your bones *now* without waiting for researchers to develop future treatments.

100. Where can I go for more information?

While many of your questions have been answered in this book, you likely will want to look for additional information on osteoporosis, osteopenia, and other health-related topics. Refer to Appendix B and the bibliography for a listing of research and resources that may be helpful as you continue to improve your overall health as well as that of your bones.

The exercises found in this appendix are reprinted from The National Institute on Aging (NIH Publication # 01-4258) *Exercise: A Guide from the National Institute on Aging,* Revised 2001.

Examples of Strength Exercises

1. Arm Raise

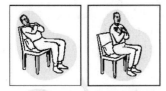

Strengthens shoulder muscles.

1. **Sit in armless chair with your back supported by back of chair.**
2. **Keep feet flat on floor spaced shoulder-width apart.**
3. **Hold hand weights straight down at your sides, with palms facing inward.**
4. **Raise both arms to side, shoulder height.**
5. **Hold the position for 1 second.**
6. **Slowly lower arms to sides. Pause.**
7. **Repeat 8 to 15 times.**
8. **Rest; then do another set of 8 to 15 repetitions.**

2. Chair Stand

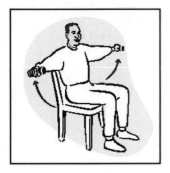

Strengthens muscles in abdomen and thighs. Your goal is to do this exercise without using your hands as you become stronger.

1. **Place pillows on the back of chair.**
2. **Sit toward front of chair, knees bent, feet flat on floor.**
3. **Lean back on pillows in half-reclining position. Keep your back and shoulders straight throughout exercise.**
4. **Raise upper body forward until sitting upright, using hands as little as possible (or not at all, if you can). Your back should no longer lean against pillows.**
5. **Slowly stand up, using hands as little as possible.**
6. **Slowly sit back down. Pause.**
7. **Repeat 8 to 15 times.**
8. **Rest; then do another set of 8 to 15 repetitions.**

3. Biceps Curl

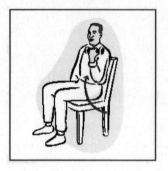

Strengthens upper-arm muscles.

1. Sit in armless chair with your back supported by back of chair.
2. Keep feet flat on floor spaced shoulder-width apart.
3. Hold hand weights straight down at your sides, with palms facing inward.
4. Slowly bend one elbow, lifting weight toward chest. (Rotate palm to face shoulder while lifting weight.)
5. Hold position for 1 second.
6. Slowly lower arm to starting position. Pause.
7. Repeat with other arm.
8. Alternate arms until you have done 8 to 15 repetitions with each arm.
9. Rest; then do another set of 8 to 15 alternating repetitions.

4. Plantar Flexion

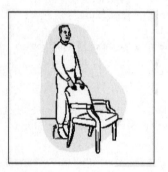

Strengthens ankle and calf muscles. Use ankle weights, if you are ready.

1. Stand straight, feet flat on floor, holding onto a table or chair for balance.
2. Slowly stand on tiptoe, as high as possible.
3. Hold position for 1 second.
4. Slowly lower heels all the way back down. Pause.
5. Do the exercise 8 to 15 times.
6. Rest; then do another set of 8 to 15 repetitions.

Variation:

As you become stronger, do the exercise standing on one leg only, alternating legs for a total of 8 to 15 times on each leg. Rest; then do another set of 8 to 15 alternating repetitions.

5. Triceps Extension

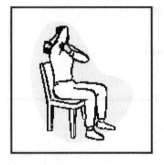

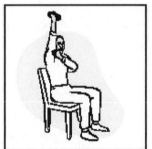

(If your shoulders aren't flexible enough to do this exercise, see alternative "Dip" exercise, No. 6.)

Strengthens muscles in back of upper arm. Keep supporting your arm with your hand throughout the exercise.

1. Sit in chair with your back supported by back of chair.
2. Keep feet flat on floor, shoulder-width apart.
3. Hold a weight in one hand. Raise that arm straight toward ceiling, palm facing in.
4. Support this arm below elbow with other hand.
5. Slowly bend raised arm at elbow, bringing hand weight toward same shoulder.
6. Slowly straighten arm toward ceiling.
7. Hold position for 1 second.
8. Slowly bend arm toward shoulder again. Pause.
9. Repeat the bending and straightening until you have done the exercise 8 to 15 times.
10. Repeat 8 to 15 times with your other arm.
11. Rest; then do another set of 8 to 15 alternating repetitions.

6. Alternative "Dip" Exercise for Back of Upper Arm

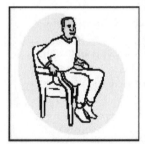

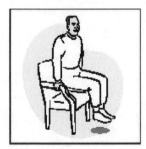

This pushing motion will strengthen your arm muscles even if you aren't yet able to lift yourself up off of the chair. Don't use your legs or feet for assistance, or use them as little as possible.

1. Sit in chair with armrests.
2. Lean slightly forward, keep your back and shoulders straight.
3. Grasp arms of chair. Your hands should be level with trunk of body or slightly farther forward.
4. Tuck feet slightly under chair, heels off the ground, weight on toes and balls of feet.
5. Slowly push body off of chair using arms, not legs.
6. Slowly lower back down to starting position. Pause.
7. Repeat 8 to 15 times.
8. Rest; then do another set of 8 to 15 repetitions.

7. Knee Flexion

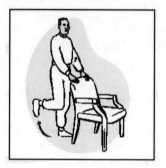

Strengthens muscles in back of thigh. Use ankle weights, if you are ready.

1. **Stand straight holding onto a table or chair for balance.**
2. **Slowly bend knee as far as possible. Don't move your upper leg at all; bend your knee only.**
3. **Hold position for 1 second.**
4. **Slowly lower foot all the way back down. Pause.**
5. **Repeat with other leg.**
6. **Alternate legs until you have done 8 to 15 repetitions with each leg.**
7. **Rest; then do another set of 8 to 15 alternating repetitions.**

8. Hip Flexion

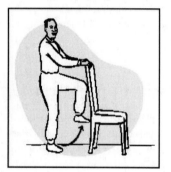

Strengthens thigh and hip muscles. Use ankle weights, if you are ready.

1. **Stand straight to the side or behind a chair or table, holding on for balance.**
2. **Slowly bend one knee toward chest, without bending waist or hips.**
3. **Hold position for 1 second.**
4. **Slowly lower leg all the way down. Pause.**
5. **Repeat with other leg.**
6. **Alternate legs until you have done 8 to 15 repetitions with each leg.**
7. **Rest; then do another set of 8 to 15 alternating repetitions.**

9. Shoulder Flexion

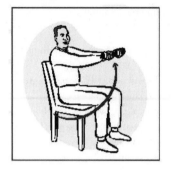

Strengthens shoulder muscles.

1. **Sit in armless chair with your back supported by back of chair.**
2. **Keep feet flat on floor even with your shoulders.**
3. **Hold hand weights straight down at your sides, with palms facing inward.**
4. **Raise both arms in front of you (keep them straight and rotate so palms face upward) to shoulder height.**
5. **Hold position for 1 second.**
6. **Slowly lower arms to sides. Pause.**
7. **Repeat 8 to 15 times.**
8. **Rest; then do another set of 8 to 15 repetitions.**

10. Knee Extension

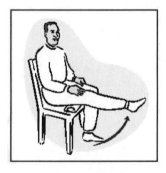

Strengthens muscles in front of thigh and shin.
Use ankle weights, if you are ready.

1. **Sit in chair. Only the balls of your feet and your toes should rest on the floor. Put rolled towel under knees, if needed, to lift your feet. Rest your hands on your thighs or on the sides of the chair.**
2. **Slowly extend one leg in front of you as straight as possible.**
3. **Flex foot to point toes toward head.**
4. **Hold position for 1 to 2 seconds.**
5. **Slowly lower leg back down. Pause.**
6. **Repeat with other leg.**
7. **Alternate legs until you have done 8 to 15 repetitions with each leg.**
8. **Rest; then do another set of 8 to 15 alternating repetitions.**

11. Hip Extension

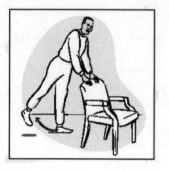

Strengthens buttock and lower-back muscles. Use ankle weights, if you are ready.

1. **Stand 12 to 18 inches from a table or chair, feet slightly apart.**
2. **Bend forward at hips at about 45-degree angle; hold onto a table or chair for balance.**
3. **Slowly lift one leg straight backwards without bending your knee, pointing your toes, or bending your upper body any farther forward.**
4. **Hold position for 1 second.**
5. **Slowly lower leg. Pause.**
6. **Repeat with other leg.**
7. **Alternate legs until you have done 8 to 15 repetitions with each leg.**
8. **Rest; then do another set of 8 to 15 alternating repetitions.**

12. Side Leg Raise

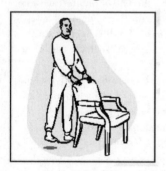

Strengthens muscles at sides of hips and thighs. Use ankle weights, if you are ready.

1. **Stand straight, directly behind table or chair, feet slightly apart.**
2. **Hold onto a table or chair for balance.**
3. **Slowly lift one leg 6–12 inches out to side. Keep your back and both legs straight. Don't point your toes outward; keep them facing forward.**
4. **Hold position for 1 second.**
5. **Slowly lower leg. Pause.**
6. **Repeat with other leg.**
7. **Alternate legs until you have done 8 to 15 repetitions with each leg.**
8. **Rest; then do another set of 8 to 15 alternating repetitions.**

Osteoporosis and Bone Health

NIH Osteoporosis and Related Bone Diseases—National Resource Center
2 AMS Circle
Bethesda, MD 20892-3676
(800) 624-BONE or (800) 624-3663
www.osteo.org

National Osteoporosis Foundation
1232 22nd Street, NW
Washington, DC 20037-1292
(202) 223-2226
www.nof.org

American Society for Bone Mineral Research
2025 M Street, NW, Suite 800
Washington, DC 20036-3309
(202) 367-1161
www.asbmr.org

Centers for Disease Control and Prevention
1600 Clifton Road
Atlanta, GA 30333
(404) 639-3311
Public Inquiries: (404) 639-3534/(800) 311-3435
www.cdc.gov/nccdphp/dnpa/bonehealth/

International Osteoporosis Foundation
73, Cours Albert-Thomas
69447 Lyon Cedex 03
France
and
5 Rue Perdtemps
1260 Nyon
Switzerland
www.osteofound.org

The Surgeon General's Report on Bone Health
Office of the Surgeon General
5600 Fishers Lane
Room 18-66
Rockville, MD 20857
www.surgeongeneral.gov/library/bonehealth/
United States Bone and Joint Decade (2002–2011)
www.usbjd.org

World Health Organization (WHO)
Avenue Appia 20
1211 Geneva 27
Switzerland
Telephone: (+ 41-22) 791-21-11
Fax: (+ 41-22) 791-3111
Telex: 415-416
Telegraph: UNISANTE GENEVA
www.who.int
FRAX algorithm available at: www.shef.ac.uk/FRAX/

Prevention of Osteoporosis in Girls

Powerful Bones, Powerful Girls
National Bone Health Campaign for Girls Ages 9 to 12
Centers for Disease Control and Prevention
www.cdc.gov/nccdphp/dnpa/bonehealth/campaign.htm

By Girls, For Girls
An online education collaboration between Smith College and
the YWCA
www.bygirlsforgirls.org/previousby4g/osteoporosis.html

Nutrition and Weight Management

American Obesity Association
1250 24th Street, NW, Suite 300
Washington, DC 20037
(202) 776-7711
www.obesity.org

Center for Nutrition Policy and Promotion
United States Department of Agriculture (USDA)
www.usda.gov/cnpp

Office of Dietary Supplements
National Institutes of Health

Bethesda, MD 20892
http://dietary-supplements.info.nih.gov/

2005 Dietary Guidelines available at:
Nutrition.gov
A Service of the National Agricultural Library, USDA
www.nutrition.gov

The 2005 Revised Food Pyramid (sponsored by the USDA)
www.mypyramid.gov

Exercise

Active Network (articles and events for your favorite physical
   activity)
www.active.com

American Academy of Orthopaedic Surgeons
6300 North River Road
Rosemont, Illinois 60018-4262
(847) 823-7186
www.aaos.org

American Council on Exercise
4851 Paramount Drive
San Diego, CA 92123
(858) 279-8227
www.acefitness.org

Division of Nutrition and Physical Activity
National Center for Chronic Disease Prevention and Health
   Promotion
Centers for Disease Control and Prevention
4770 Buford Highway, NE, MS/K-24
Atlanta, GA 30341-3717
(770) 488-5820
www.cdc.gov/nccdphp/dnpa/

The Healthier US Initiative
The U.S. Department of Health and Human Services
200 Independence Avenue, SW
Washington, DC 20201
(202) 619-0257
www.healthierus.gov

President's Council on Physical Fitness and Sports
Department W
200 Independence Ave SW
Room 738-H
Washington, DC 20201
(202) 690-9000
www.fitness.gov

Shape Up America and the 10,000 Steps Program
www.shapeup.org

Paget's Disease

The Paget Foundation
120 Wall Street, Suite 1602
New York, NY 10005-4001
(212) 509-5335
(800) 23-PAGET
www.paget.org

Diseases and Conditions Associated with Osteoporosis

American Association of Clinical Endocrinologists
1000 Riverside Avenue, Suite 205
Jacksonville, FL 32204
(904) 353-7878
www.aace.com

American Diabetes Association
National Call Center
1701 North Beauregard Street
Alexandria, VA 22311
800-DIABETES (800-342-2383)
www.diabetes.org

American Lung Association
61 Broadway, 6th floor
New York, NY 10006
(212) 315-8700
www.lungusa.org

Arthritis Foundation
PO Box 7669
Atlanta, GA 30357-0669
(404)872-7100/(800) 568-4045
www.arthritis.org

Crohn's & Colitis Foundation of America
386 Park Avenue South
New York, NY 10016-8804
(800) 932-2423
www.ccfa.org

Lupus Foundation of America, Inc.
2000 L Street, NW, Suite 710
Washington, DC 20036
(202) 349-1155
www.lupus.org

National Eating Disorders Association (NEDA)
603 Stewart Street, Suite 803
Seattle, WA 98101
(800) 931-2237
www.nationaleatingdisorders.org

National Institute of Diabetes, Digestive and Kidney Diseases
Of the National Institutes of Health
NIH, Building 31, Room 9A04
31 Center Drive, MSC 2560
Bethesda, MD 20892-2560
www.niddk.nih.gov/

Menopause and Women's Health

American College of Nurse-Midwives
818 Connecticut Avenue NW, Suite 900
Washington, DC 20006
(202) 728-9860
www.midwife.org

American College of Obstetricians and Gynecologists
409 12th Street, SW, PO Box 96920
Washington, DC 20090-6920
(202) 863-2518 (patient information brochures)
www.acog.org

Breast Cancer Education Web Site
111 Forrest Avenue 1R
Narberth, PA 19072
www.breastcancer.org

National Asian Women's Health Organization
One Embarcadero Center, Suite 500
San Francisco, CA 94111
(415) 773-2838
www.nawho.org

**National Association of Nurse Practitioners
in Women's Health**
505 C Street, NE
Washington, DC 20002
(202) 543-9693
www.npwh.org

National Women's Health Information Center
United States Department of Health and
  Human Services
(800) 994-9662
www.4women.gov

National Women's Health Resource Center
157 Broad Street, Suite 315
Red Bank, NJ 07701
(877) 986-9472/Fax: (732) 530-3347
info@healthywomen.org
www.healthywomen.org

North American Menopause Society (NAMS)
PO Box 94527
Cleveland, OH 44101
(440) 442-7550
www.menopause.org

Power-Surge, An Online Menopause Community
www.power-surge.com

Women's Health Initiative
National Heart Lung and Blood Institute
NHLBI Health Information Center
PO Box 30105
Bethesda, MD 20824-0105
(301) 592-8573
www.nhlbi.nih.gov/whi/

Clinical Trials

Clinical Trials: A Service of the National Institutes of Health
  (linking patients to medical research)
www.clinicaltrials.gov

General Health

Centers for Disease Control and Prevention (CDC)
1600 Clifton Road
Atlanta, GA 30333
(800) 311-3435
www.cdc.gov

ivillage.com
www.ivillage.com

Mayo Clinic Health Information
www.mayoclinic.com

National Institute on Aging
National Information Center
PO Box 8057
Gaithersburg, MD 20898
(800) 222-2225
www.nia.nih.gov

National Library of Medicine (Health Information)
National Institutes of Health
Medline Plus
http://medlineplus.gov/

Complementary and Alternative Therapies

Acupuncture Resources for Patients
www.acupuncture.com

American Botanical Council
www.herbalgram.org

American Massage Therapy Association
820 Davis Street
Evanston, IL 60201
www.amtamassage.org

ConsumerLab.com
(evaluates quality of herbs, vitamins, dietary and nutritional
   supplements)
ConsumerLab.com, LLC
333 Mamaroneck Avenue
White Plains, NY 10605
(914) 722-9149
www.consumerlab.com

National Center for Complementary and Alternative Medicine (NCCAM)
PO Box 7923
Gaithersburg, MD 20898
(888) 644-6226
www.nccam.nih.gov

Natural Medicines Comprehensive Database
(begun in 1999 and updated daily, this site provides an evaluation
   by 50 clinical pharmacists and physicians for a comprehensive
   listing of brand-name products and their ingredients)
www.naturaldatabase.com

Mental Health, Depression, and Social Isolation

Girlfriends for Life
www.girlfriendsforlife.org

**National Institute of Mental
Health (NIMH)**
Office of Communications
6001 Executive Boulevard, Room 8184, MSC 9663
Bethesda, MD 20892-9663
(866) 615-6464
www.nimh.nih.gov

The Red Hat Society
Fun and Friendship After Age 50
www.redhatsociety.com

Compounding Pharmacies

Women's International Pharmacy
(800) 279-5708
www.womensinternational.com

Directory of Compounding Pharmacies
http://dmoz.org/Health/Pharmacy/Pharmacies/Compounding/

Hip Protectors, Fall Prevention Devices, and Medication Reminders

e-pill, LLC
70 Walnut Street
Wellesley, MA 02481
(800) 930-9255
www.HIProtector.com

Listing of Contents of Common Antacids

National Library of Medicine
www.nlm.nih.gov/medlineplus/druginfo/uspdi/202047.html#GX
   Xg20204715

Smoking Cessation

Cessation Resource Center
Office on Smoking and Health
NCCDPHP/CDC
Mail Stop K-50
4770 Buford Highway, NE
Atlanta, GA 30341-3717
(800) CDC-1311
http://apps.nccd.cdc.gov/crc/

U.S. Department of Health and Human Services
200 Independence Avenue, SW
Washington, DC 20201
www.surgeongeneral.gov/tobacco/

Bibliography

In addition to the resources listed earlier, the following publications and scientific sources were used as references in the preparation of this book. Abstracts for most of these articles are available free on the National Library of Medicine's Web Site, PubMed (www.ncbi.nlm.nih.gov/entrez/query.fcgi?DB=pubmed), and complete articles can be downloaded for a nominal fee.

Akkus O, Polyakova-Akkus A, Adar F, Schaffler MB. Aging of microstructural compartments in human compact bone. *J Bone Miner Res* Jun 2003;18(6):1012–1019.

American Association of Oral and Maxillofacial Surgeons. AAOMS position paper on bisphosphonate-related osteonecrosis of the jaw. http://www.aaoms.org/docs/position_papers/osteonecrosis.pdf. Published September 26, 2006. Accessed May 22, 2009.

American Cancer Society. Cancer Statistics 2004. *ACS*. Available at: www.cancer.org. Accessed August 2005.

American College of Rheumatology. Recommendations for the prevention and treatment of GIO. *Arthritis Rheum* 2001;44:1496–1503.

American Heart Association. *Heart Disease and Stroke Statistics—2003 Update*. Dallas, TX: American Heart Association; 2003.

American Association of Clinical Endocrinologists. Medical guidelines for clinical practice for the prevention and treatment of postmenopausal osteoporosis. *Endocr Pract* 2003;9:544–564.

Anonymous. eHippocrates. Updated daily, 2009, Accessed September 28, 2009.

Atkinson C, Compston JE, Day NE, et al. The effects of phyto-estrogen isoflavones on bone density in women: a double-blind, randomized, placebo-controlled trial. *Am J Clin Nutr* 2004;79:326–333.

Atkinson C, Warren RM, Sala E, et al. Red-clover-derived isoflavones and mammographic breast density: a double-blind, randomized, placebo-controlled trial. *Breast Cancer Res* 2004;6:R170–R179.

Bagger YZ, Tanko LB, Alexandersen P, et al. Two to three years of hormone replacement treatment in healthy women have long-term preventive effects on bone mass and osteoporotic fractures: the PERF study. *Bone* Apr 2004;34(4):728–735.

Balzini L, Vannucchi L, Benvenuti F, et al. Clinical characteristics of flexed posture in elderly women. *J Am Geriatr Soc* 2003;51:1419–1426.

Barnes PM, Powell-Griner E, McFann K, Nahin RL. *Complementary and Alternative Medicine Use Among Adults: United States, 2002.* Washington, DC: CDC Advance Data Report #343; 2002.

Baron JA, Beach M, Wallace K, et al. Risk of prostate cancer in a randomized clinical trial of calcium supplementation. *Cancer Epidemiol Biomarkers Prev* 2005;14:586–589.

Barrett-Connor E, Mosca L, Collins P, et al. Effects of raloxifene on cardiovascular events and breast cancer in postmenopausal women. *N Engl J Med* Jul 13 2006;355(2):125–137.

Bauer DC, Mundy GR, Jamal SA, et al. Use of statins and fracture: results of 4 prospective studies and cumulative meta-analysis of observational studies and controlled trials. *Arch Intern Med* 2004;164:146–152.

Benjamin HJ, Glow KM. Strength training for children and adolescents. *Physician Sportsmed* 2003:31(9). Available at: www.physsportsmed.com/issues/2003/0903/benjamin.htm. Accessed August 2005.

Beral V. Breast cancer and hormone-replacement therapy in the Million Women Study. *Lancet* 2003;362:419–427.

Bertone-Johnson ER, Hankinson SE, Bendich A, et al. Calcium and vitamin D intake and risk of incident premenstrual syndrome. *Arch Intern Med* 2005;165:1246–1252.

Appendix B

Bilezikian JP. Osteonecrosis of the jaw—do bisphosphonates pose a risk? *N Engl J Med* Nov 30 2006;355(22):2278–2281.

Binkley NC, Schmeer P, Wasnich RD, Lenchik L. What are the criteria by which a densitometric diagnosis of osteoporosis can be made in males and non-Caucasians? *J Clin Densitom* 2002;5(Suppl):S19–S27.

Birks Y. A structured education programme increased hip protector use and may reduce hip fractures in nursing homes. *Evid Based Nurs* 2003;6:114–115.

Birks YF, Hildreth R, Campbell P, et al. Randomised controlled trial of hip protectors for the prevention of second hip fractures. *Age Ageing* 2003;32:442–444.

Birks YF, Porthouse J, Addie C, et al. Randomized controlled trial of hip protectors among women living in the community. *Osteoporos Int* 2004;15:701–706.

Bischoff-Ferrari HA, Dietrich T, Orav EJ, et al. Higher 25-hydroxyvitamin D concentrations are associated with better lower-extremity function in both active and inactive persons aged > or =60 y. *Am J Clin Nutr* 2004;80:752–758.

Black DM, Bilezikian JP, Ensrud KE, et al. One year of alendronate after one year of parathyroid hormone (1–84) for osteoporosis. *N Engl J Med* Aug 11 2005;353(6):555–565.

Black DM, Greenspan SL, Ensrud KF, et al. The effects of parathyroid hormone and alendronate alone or in combination in postmenopausal osteoporosis. *N Engl J Med* 2003; 249(13):1207–1215.

Black DM, Schwartz AV, Ensrud KE, et al. Effects of continuing or stopping alendronate after 5 years of treatment: the Fracture Intervention Trial Long-term Extension (FLEX): a randomized trial. *JAMA* Dec 27 2006;296(24):2927–2938.

Black DM, Thompson DE, Bauer DC, et al. Fracture risk reduction with alendronate in women with osteoporosis: the Fracture Intervention Trial. FIT Research Group. *J Clin Endocrinol Metab* 2000;85:4118–4124.

Bobrow RS. Thiazide use and reduced sodium intake for prevention of osteoporosis. *JAMA* 2001;285:2323; author reply, 2324.

Boivin G, Meunier PJ. Changes in bone remodeling rate influence the degree of mineralization of bone. *Connect Tissue Res* 2002;43(2–3):535–537.

Bolland M, Hay D, Grey A, Reid I, Cundy T. Osteonecrosis of the jaw and bisphosphonates—putting the risk in perspective. *N Z Med J* 2006;119(1246):U2339.

Bolognese M, Krege JH, Utian WH, et al. Effects of arzoxifene on bone mineral density and endometrium in postmenopausal women with normal or low bone mass. *J Clin Endocrinol Metab* Jul 2009;94(7):2284–2289.

Bone HG, Greenspan SL, McKeever C, et al. Alendronate and estrogen effects in postmenopausal women with low bone mineral density. Alendronate/Estrogen Study Group. *J Clin Endocrinol Metab* Feb 2000;85(2): 720–726.

Bone HG, Hosking D, Devogelaer J-P, et al. Ten years' experience with alendronate for osteoporosis in postmenopausal women. *N Engl J Med* 2004;350:1189–1199.

Campbell WW, Crim MC, Young VR, Evans WJ. Increased energy requirements and changes in body composition with resistance training in older adults. *Am J Clin Nutr* 1994;60:167–175.

Carbone LD, Nevitt MC, Wildy K, et al. The relationship of antiresorptive drug use to structural findings and symptoms of knee osteoarthritis. *Arthritis Rheum* 2004;50:3516–3525.

Cauley JA, Lui LY, Ensrud KE, et al. Bone mineral density and the risk of incident nonspinal fractures in black and white women. *JAMA* 2005;293:2102–2108.

Cauley JA, Robbins J, Chen Z, et al. Effects of estrogen plus progestin on risk of fracture and bone mineral density: the Women's Health Initiative randomized trial. *JAMA* 2003;290:1729–1738.

Chan K, Qin L, Lau M, et al. A randomized, prospective study of the effects of Tai Chi Chun exercise on bone mineral density in postmenopausal women. *Arch Phys Med Rehabil* 2004;85:717–722.

Chen Z, Ettinger MB, Ritenbaugh C, et al. Habitual tea consumption and risk of osteoporosis: a prospective study in the Women's Health Initiative Observational Cohort. *Am J Epidemiol* 2003:158:772–781.

Chesnut CH 3rd, Bell NH, Clark GS, et al. Hormone replacement therapy in postmenopausal women: urinary N-telopeptide of type I collagen monitors therapeutic effect and predicts response of bone mineral density. *Am J Med* 1997;102:29–37.

Chesnut CH 3rd, Silverman S, Andriano K, et al. A randomized trial of nasal spray salmon calcitonin in postmenopausal women with established osteoporosis: the prevent recurrence of osteoporotic fractures study. PROOF Study Group. *Am J Med* 2000;109:267–276.

Appendix B

Ciarella TE, Fyhrie DP, Parfitt AM. Effects of vertebral bone fragility and bone formation rate on the mineralization levels of cancellous bone from white females. *Bone* 2003;32:311–315.

Cizza G, Ravn P, Chrousos GP, Gold PW. Depression: a major, unrecognized risk factor for osteoporosis? *Trends Endocrinol Metab* 2001;12(5):198–203.

Clifton-Bligh PB, Baber RJ, Fulcher GR, et al. The effect of isoflavones extracted from red clover (Rimostil) on lipid and bone metabolism). *Menopause* 2001;8:259–265.

Clyman B. Exercise in the treatment of osteoarthritis. *Curr Rheumatol Rep* 2001;3:520–523.

Coelho R, Silva C, Maia A, Prata J, Barros H. Bone mineral density and depression: a community study in women. *J Psychosom Res* 1999;46(1):29–35.

Cohen L. Depression rates in perimenopausal and premenopausal women: a longitudinal study (abstract). American Psychiatric Association Annual Meeting, New York, NY; April, 2004.

Col NF, Eckman MH, Karas RH, et al. Patient-specific decisions about hormone replacement therapy in postmenopausal women. *JAMA* 1997;277:1140–1147.

Coleman RE. Optimising treatment of bone metastases by Aredia™ and Zometa™. *Breast Cancer* 2000;7:361–369.

Colon-Emeric CS, Caminis J, Suh TT, et al. The HORIZON Recurrent Fracture Trial: design of a clinical trial in the prevention of subsequent fractures after low trauma hip fracture repair. *Curr Med Res Opin* 2004;20:903–910.

Cook AJ, Friday JE. Food mixture or ingredient sources for dietary calcium: shifts in food group contributions using four grouping protocols. *J Am Dietetic Assoc* 2003;103(11):1513–1519.

Cooper C, Atkinson EJ, Jacobsen SJ, et al. Population-based study of survival after osteoporotic fractures. *Am J Epidemiol* 1993;137:1001–1005.

Cramer JA, Monkar MM, Hebborn A, Suppaganya A. Does dosing regimen impact persistence with bisphosphonate therapy among postmenopausal osteoporotic women? (poster #M434). Presented at: 26th Annual Meeting of the American Society for Bone Mineral Research; October 1–5, 2004, 2004; Seattle, WA.

Creditor MC. Hazards of hospitalization of the elderly. *Ann Intern Med* Feb 1 1993;118(3):219–223.

Cromer BA, Lazebnik R, Rome E, et al. Double-blinded randomized controlled trial of estrogen supplementation in adolescent girls who receive depot medroxyprogesterone acetate for contraception. *Am J Obstet Gynecol* 2005;192:42–47.

Cummings SR, Browner WS, Bauer D, et al. Endogenous hormones and the risk of hip and vertebral fractures among older women. Study of Osteoporotic Fractures Research Group. *N Engl J Med* 1998;339:733–738.

Cummings SR, Eckert S, Krueger KA, et al. The effect of raloxifene on risk of breast cancer in postmenopausal women: results from the MORE randomized trial. Multiple Outcomes of Raloxifene Evaluation. *JAMA* 1999;281:2189–2197.

Cummings SR, Ettinger B, Delmas PD, et al. for the LIFT Trial investigators. The effects of tibolone in older postmenopausal women. *N Engl J Med* 2008:359:697–708.

Cummings SR, Melton LJ. Epidemiology and outcomes of osteoporotic fractures. *Lancet* 2002;359:1761–1767.

Cummings SR, Nevitt MC, Browner WS, et al. Risk factors for hip fracture in white women. Study of Osteoporotic Fractures Research Group. *N Engl J Med* 1995;332:767–773.

Dalsky PG, Stocke KS, Ehsani AA, et al. Weight bearing exercise training and lumbar bone mineral content in postmenopausal women. *Ann Intern Med* 1988;108:824–838.

Dawson-Hughes B, Gold DT, Rodbard HW, et al. *Physician's Guide to Prevention and Treatment of Osteoporosis*, 2nd ed. Washington, DC: National Osteoporosis Foundation; 2003.

Dawson-Hughes B, Lindsay R, Khosla S, et al. *Clinician's Guide to Prevention and Treatment of Osteoporosis*. Washington DC: National Osteoporosis Foundation; 2008; available at: http://www.nof.org/professionals/clinicians_Guide.htm Accessed September 29, 2009.

Dawson-Hughes B, Tosteson AN, Melton LJ 3rd, et al. Implications of absolute fracture risk assessment for osteoporosis practice guidelines in the USA. *Osteoporos Int* Feb 22 2008;19(4): 449–458.

Dawson-Hughes B. Racial/ethnic considerations in making recommendations for vitamin D for adult and elderly men and women. *Am J Clin Nutr* 2004;80(Suppl 6):1763S–1766S.

Delmas PD, Bjarnason NH, Mitlak BH, et al. Effects of raloxifene on bone mineral density, serum cholesterol concentrations, and uterine endometrium in postmenopausal women. *N Engl J Med* 1997;337:1641–1647.

Delmas PD, McClung MR, Zanchetta JR, et al. Efficacy and safety of risedronate 150 mg once a month in the treatment of postmenopausal osteoporosis. *Bone* Jan 2008;42(1):36–42.

Appendix B

Denosumab information on the Amgen Web Site: www.amgen.com Accessed July 6, 2009.

Deshmane V, Krishnamurthy S, Melemed AS, Peterson P, Buzdar AU. Phase III double-blind trial of arzoxifene compared with tamoxifen for locally advanced or metastatic breast cancer. *J Clin Oncol* Nov 1 2007;25(31):4967–4973.

Donangelo CM. Calcium and osteoporosis. *Arch Latinoam Nutr* Jun 1997;47(2 Suppl 1):13–16.

Ellis GK, Bone HG, Chlebowski R, et al. Randomized trial of denosumab in patients receiving adjuvant aromatase inhibitors for nonmetastatic breast cancer. *J Clin Oncol* Oct 2008;26(30): 4875–4882.

Ensrud KE, Barrett-Connor EL, Schwarts A, et al. Randomized trial of effect of alendronate continuous versus discontinuation in women with low BMD: results from the Fracture Prevention Trial long-term extension. *J Bone Min Res* 2004;19:1259–1269.

Ensrud KE, Black DM, Harris F, et al. Correlates of kyphosis in older women. The Fracture Intervention Trial Research Group. *J Am Geriatr Soc* 1997;45:682–687.

Ensrud KE, Cauley J, Lipschutz R, Cummings SR. Weight change and fractures in older women. Study of Osteoporotic Fractures Research Group. *Arch Intern Med* 1997;157:857–863.

Ensrud KE, Ewing SK, Stone KL, et al. Intentional and unintentional weight loss, increased bone loss and hip fracture risk in older women. *J Am Geriatr Soc* 2003;51:1740–1747.

Ensrud KE, Fullman RL, Barrett-Connor E, et al. Voluntary weight reduction in older men increases hip bone loss: the Osteoporotic Fractures in Men study. *J Clin Endocrinol Metab* 2005;90:1998–2004.

Ettinger B, Ensrud KE, Wallace R, et al. Effects of ultralow-dose transdermal estradiol on bone mineral density: a randomized clinical trial. *Obstet Gynecol* Sep 2004;104(3):443–451.

Ettinger B, San Martin J, Crans G, Pavo I. Differential effects of teriparatide on BMD after treatment with raloxifene or alendronate. *J Bone Miner Res* 2004;19:745–751.

Farmer ME, Harris T, Madans JH, et al. Anthropometric indicators and hip fracture. The NHANES I epidemiologic follow-up study. *J Am Geriatr Soc* 1989;37:9–16.

Feltes C, Fountas KN, Machinis T, et al. Immediate and early postoperative pain relief after kyphoplasty without significant restoration of vertebral body height in acute osteoporotic vertebral fractures. *Neurosurg Focus* 2005;18:e5.

Ferrari SL, Deutsch S, Choudhury U, et al. Polymorphisms in the low-density lipoprotein receptor-related protein 5 (*LRP5*) gene are associated with variation in vertebral bone mass, vertebral bone size, and stature in whites. *Am J Hum Genet* 2004;74:866–875.

Feskanich D, Weber P, Willett WC, et al. Vitamin K intake and hip fractures in women: a prospective study. *Am J Clin Nutr* 1999;69:74–79.

Feskanich D, Willett W, Colditz G. Walking and leisure-time activity and risk of hip fracture in postmenopausal women. *JAMA* 2002;288:2300–2306.

Finkelstein JS, Hayes A, Hunzelman JL, et al. The effects of parathyroid hormone, alendronate, or both in men with osteoporosis. *N Engl J Med* 2003;349:1216–1226.

Fitzpatrick L, Heaney RP. Got soda? *J Bone Miner Res* 2003;18:1570–1572.

Fletcher RH, Fairfield KM. Vitamins for chronic disease prevention in adults: clinical applications. *JAMA* 2002;287:3127–3129.

Fontana L, Shew JL, Holloszy JO, Villareal DT. Low bone mass in subjects on a long-term raw vegetarian diet. *Arch Intern Med* 2005;165(6): 684–9.

Forman JP, Rimm EB, Stampfer MJ, Curhan GC. Folate intake and the risk of incident hypertension among US women. *JAMA* 2005;293:320–329.

Fosteum Product. Prescription product for osteopenia and osteoporosis. Fosteum Web Site: http://www.fosteum.com. Accessed May 22, 2009.

Garnero P, Hausherr E, Chapuy MC, et al. Markers of bone resorption predict hip fracture in elderly women: the EPIDOS Prospective Study. *J Bone Miner Res* 1996;11:1531–1538.

Garnero P, Shih WJ, Gineyts E, et al. Comparison of new biochemical markers of bone turnover in late postmenopausal osteoporotic women in response to alendronate treatment. *J Clin Endocrinol Metab* 1994;79:1693–1700.

Giovannucci E. The epidemiology of vitamin D and cancer incidence and mortality: a review (United States). *Cancer Causes Control* 2005;16:83–95.

Gluck OS, Maricic MJ, Leib ES, Lewiecki EM. Recommendations regarding individuals in whom bone densitometry should be performed: comment on the article by van Staa et al. *Arthritis Rheum* 2004;50:2715–2716.

Appendix B

Gold DT, Lee LS, Tresolini CP, eds. *Working with Patients to Prevent, Treat, and Manage Osteoporosis: A Curriculum Guide for the Health Professions, 3rd ed.* Available at www.geri.duke.edu/pepper/osteocurriculum/index.html. Durham, NC: Center for the Study of Aging and Human Development, Duke University Medical Center; 2001.

Grady D, Ettinger B, Moscarelli E, et al. Safety and adverse effects associated with raloxifene: multiple outcomes of raloxifene evaluation. *Obstet Gynecol* Oct 2004;104(4):837–844.

Greendale GA, Barrett-Connor E. Outcomes of osteoporotic fractures. In: Marcus R, Feldman D, Kelsey J, eds. *Osteoporosis*, 2nd ed. San Diego, CA: Academic Press; 2001:819–829.

Greenspan SL, Emkey RD, Bone HG, et al. Significant differential effects of alendronate, estrogen, or combination therapy on the rate of bone loss after discontinuation of treatment of postmenopausal osteoporosis. A randomized, double-blind, placebo-controlled trial. *Ann Intern Med* 2002;137: 875–883.

Greenspan SL, Resnick NM, Parker RA. Combination therapy with hormone replacement and alendronate for prevention of bone loss in elderly women: a randomized controlled trial. *JAMA* 2003;289:2525–2533.

Guillaume G. Postmenopausal osteoporosis and Chinese medicine. *Am J Acupunct* 1992;20:105–111.

Hall SE, Criddle RA, Comito TL, Prince RL. A case-control study of quality of life and functional impairment in women with long-standing vertebral osteoporotic fracture. *Osteoporos Int* 1999;9:508–515.

Hamdy RC, Petak SM, Lenchik L. Which central dual X-ray absorptiometry skeletal sites and regions of interest should be used to determine the diagnosis of osteoporosis? *J Clin Densitom* 2002;5(Suppl):S11–S18.

Hanley DA, Ioannidis G, Adachi JD. Etridronate therapy in the treatment and prevention of osteoporosis. *J Clin Densitom* 2000;3:79–95.

Harris ST, Eriksen EF, Davidson M, et al. Effect of combined risedronate and hormone replacement therapies on bone mineral density in postmenopausal women. *J Clin Endocrinol Metab* 2001;86:1890–1897.

Harvard Medical School. *The Benefits and Risks of Vitamins and Minerals: What You Need to Know.* Boston, MA: Harvard Medical School-Harvard Health Publications; 2003.

Hayden JA, van Tulder MW, Malmivaara AV, Koes BW. Meta-analysis: exercise therapy for nonspecific low back pain. *Ann Intern Med* 2005;142:765–775.

Hayden JA, van Tulder MW, Tomlinson G. Systematic review: strategies for using exercise therapy to improve outcomes in chronic low back pain. *Ann Intern Med* 2005;142:776–785.

Hochberg MC, Greenspan S, Wasnich RD, et al. Changes in bone density and turnover explain the reductions in incidence of nonvertebral fractures that occur during treatment with antiresorptive agents. *J Clin Endocrinol Metab* 2002;87:1586–1592.

Hodgson SF, Watts SF. American Association of Clinical Endocrinologists medical guidelines for clinical practice for the prevention and treatment of postmenopausal osteoporosis: 2001 edition with selected updates for 2003. *Endocr Pract* 2003 2003;9:544–564.

Hoerger TJ, Downs KE, Lakshmanan MC, et al. Healthcare use among U.S. women aged 45 and older: total costs and costs for selected postmenopausal health risks. *J Womens Health Gend Based Med* 1999;8:1077–1089.

Institute of Medicine. *Dietary Reference Intakes for Calcium, Phosphorus, Magnesium, Vitamin D, and Fluoride*. Washington, DC: National Academy Press; 1997.

Jeffcoat MK, Lewis CE, Reddy MS, et al. Post-menopausal bone loss and its relationship to oral bone loss. *Periodontology* 2000;23:94–102.

Johnell O, Scheele WH, Lu Y, et al. Additive effects of raloxifene and alendronate on bone density and biochemical markers of bone remodeling in postmenopausal women with osteoporosis. *J Clin Endocrinol Metab* 2002;87:985–992.

Kalkwarf HJ, Specker BL. Bone mineral changes during pregnancy and lactation. *Endocrine* 2002;17:49–53.

Kanis JA, Black D, Cooper C, et al. A new approach to the development of assessment guidelines for osteoporosis. *Osteoporos Int* 2002;13:527–536.

Kanis JA. Diagnosis of osteoporosis and assessment of fracture risk. *Lancet* 2002;359:1929–1936.

Kerstetter JE, O'Brien KO, Insogna KL. Low protein intake: the impact on calcium and bone homeostasis in humans. *J Nutr* 2003;133:855S–861S.

Khan AA, Bachrach L, Brown JP, et al. Standards and guidelines for performing central dual-energy x-ray absorptiometry in

Appendix B

premenopausal women, men, and children. *J Clin Densitom* 2004;7:51–64.

Kiel D. Hip protectors. Paper presented at: The Surgeon General's Workshop on Osteoporosis and Bone Health; Dec 12-13, 2002; Washington, DC.

Kiel DP, Felson DT, Hannan MT, et al. Caffeine and the risk of hip fracture: the Framingham Study. *Am J Epidemiol* 1990;132:675–684.

Kostenuik PJ, Capparelli C, Morony S, et al. OPG and PTH-(1-34) have additive effects on bone density and mechanical strength in osteopenic ovariectomized rats. *Endocrinology* 2001;142:4295–4304.

Kristal AR, Littman AJ, Benitez D, White E. Yoga practice is associated with attenuated weight gain in healthy, middle-aged men and women. *Altern Ther Health Med* 2005;11(4):28–33.

Krolner B, Toft B. Vertebral bone loss: an unheeded side effect of therapeutic bed rest. *Clin Sci (Lond)* 1983;64(5):537–540.

Lambing CL. Osteoporosis prevention, detection, and treatment. A mandate for primary care physicians. *Postgrad Med* Jun 2000;107(7):37–41, 44, 47–38 passim.

Landman JO, Hamdy NA, Pauwels EK, Papapoulos SE. Skeletal metabolism in patients with osteoporosis after discontinuation of long term treatment with oral pamidronate. *J Clin Endocrinol Metab* 1995;80:3465–3468.

Lanou AJ, Berkow SE, Barnard ND. Calcium, dairy products, and bone health in children and young adults: a reevaluation of the evidence. *Pediatrics* 2005;115:736–743.

Leib ES, Lewiecki EM, Binkley N, Hamdy RC. Official positions of the International Society for Clinical Densitometry. *J Clin Densitom* 2004;7:1–6.

Lewiecki EM. Bazedoxifene and bazedoxifene combined with conjugated estrogens for the management of postmenopausal osteoporosis. *Expert Opin Investig Drugs* Oct 2007;16(10): 1663–1672.

Lewiecki EM. Emerging drugs for postmenopausal osteoporosis. Expert Opin. *Emerging Drugs* 2009; 14(1):129–144.

Lindsay R, Cosman F, Lobo RA, Walsh BW, Harris ST, Reagan JE, Liss CL, Melton ME, Byrnes CA Addition of alendronate to ongoing hormone replacement therapy in the treatment of osteoporosis: a randomized, controlled clinical trial. *J Clin Endocrinol Metab* 1999;84:3076–3081.

Lindsay R, Silverman SL, Cooper C, et al. Risk of new vertebral fracture in the year following a fracture. *JAMA* 2001;285:320–323.

Lloyd T, Johnson-Rollings N, Eggli D, et al. Bone status among postmenopausal women with different habitual caffeine intakes: a longitudinal investigation. *J Am Coll Nutr* 2000; 19(2):256–261.

Looker AC, Orwoll ES, Johnston CC Jr, et al. Prevalence of low femoral bone density in older U.S. adults from NHANES III. *J Bone Miner Res* 1997;12:1761–1768.

Looker AC, Wahner HW, Dunn WL, et al. Updated data on proximal femur bone mineral levels of US adults. *Osteopor Int* 1998;8:468–489.

Lyles KW, Colon-Emeric CS, Magaziner JS, et al. Zoledronic acid and clinical fractures and mortality after hip fracture. *N Engl J Med* Nov 1 2007;357(18):1799-1809.

Lyles KW, Colon-Emeric CS, Magaziner JS, et al. Zoledronic acid in reducing clinical fracture and mortality after hip fracture. *N Engl J Med* 2007;357:nihpa40967.

Magaziner J, Hawkes W, Hebel JR, et al. Recovery from hip fracture in eight areas of function. *J Gerontol A Biol Sci Med Sci* 2000;55:M498–M507.

Majumdar SR, Kim N, Colman I, et al. Incidental vertebral fractures discovered with chest radiography in the emergency department: prevalence, recognition, and osteoporosis management in a cohort of elderly patients. *Arch Intern Med* 2005;165:905–909.

McClung MR, Lewiecki EM, Cohen SB, et al. Denosumab in postmenopausal women with low bone mineral density. *N Engl J Med* Feb 2006;354(8):821–831.

McClung MR, San Martin J, Miller PD, et al. Opposite bone remodeling effects of teriparatide and alendronate in increasing bone mass. *Arch Intern Med* 2005;165:1762–1768.

McClung MR, Wasnich RD, Hosking DJ, et al. Prevention of postmenopausal bone loss: six-year results from the early postmenopausal intervention cohort study. *J Clin Endocrinol Metab* 2004;89:4879–4885.

McClung MR, Wasnich RD, Recker R, et al. Oral daily ibandronate prevents bone loss in early postmenopausal women without osteoporosis. *J Bone Miner Res* 2004;19:11–18.

McClung MR. Osteonecrosis of the jaw. *Menopause e-Consult.* April 2007;3(2).

McLean RR, Jacques PF, Selhub J, et al. Homocysteine as a predictive factor for hip fracture in older persons. *N Engl J Med* 2004;350:2042–2049.

Mease PJ, Ginzler EM, Gluck OS, et al. Effects of prasterone on bone mineral density in women with systemic lupus erythematosus receiving chronic glucocorticoid therapy. *J Rheumatol* 2005;32:616–621.

Mehta NM, Malootian A, Gilligan JP. Calcitonin for osteoporosis and bone pain. *Curr Pharm Des* 2003;9:2659–2676.

Melton LJ 3rd, Chrischilles EA, Cooper C, et al. Perspective. How many women have osteoporosis? *J Bone Miner Res* 1992;7:1005–1010.

Melton LJ 3rd, Khosla S, Achenbach SJ, et al. Effects of body size and skeletal site on the estimated prevalence of osteoporosis in women and men. *Osteopor Int* 2000;11:977–983.

Meunier PJ, Delmas PD, Eastell R, et al. Diagnosis and management of osteoporosis in postmenopausal women: clinical guidelines. International Committee for Osteoporosis Clinical Guidelines. *Clin Ther* 1999;21:1025–1044.

Meyer G, Warnke A, Bender R, Muhlhauser I. Effect on hip fractures of increased use of hip protectors in nursing homes: cluster randomised controlled trial. *BMJ* 2003;326:76.

Michel BA, Lane NE, Bjorkengren A, et al. Impact of running on lumbar bone density: a 5-year longitudinal study. *J Rheumatol* 1992;19:1759–1763.

Michelson D, Stratakis C, Hill L, Reynolds J, Galliven E, Chrousos G, Gold P. Bone mineral density in women with depression. *N Engl J Med* 1996; 335(16): 1176–1181.

Miller PD, Bonnick SL, Johnston CC, et al. The challenges of peripheral bone density testing: which patients need additional central density skeletal measurements? *J Clin Densitom* 1998;1:211–217.

Miller PD, Watts NB, Licata AA, et al. Cyclical etidronate in the treatment of postmenopausal osteoporosis: efficacy and safety after seven years of treatment. *Am J Med* 1997;103:468–476.

Mortensen L, Charles P, Bekker PJ, et al. Risedronate increases bone mass in an early postmenopausal population: two years of treatment plus one year of follow-up. *J Clin Endocrinol Metab* 1998;83:396–402.

Munger KL, Zhang SM, O'Reilly E, et al. Vitamin D intake and incidence of multiple sclerosis. *Neurology* 2004;62:60–65.

National Institutes of Health. Osteoporosis and African American Women. *Osteoporosis and Related Bone Diseases-National Resources Center*, Revised 1/1/2003. Available at www.osteo.org/newfile.asp?doc=r607i&doctype=HTML+Fact +Sheet&doctitle=Osteoporosis+and+African%2DAmerican+ Women. Accessed August 2005.

National Library of Medicine, Web Site for Clinical Trials, Effects of arzoxifene on bone fractures and incidence of breast cancer, http://clinicaltrials.gov/ct2/show/NCT00088010. Accessed July 23, 2009.

Nelson HD, Morris CD, Kraemer DF, et al. *Osteoporosis in Postmenopausal Women: Diagnosis and Monitoring Evidence Report/Technology Assessment No. 28.* Rockville, MD: Agency for Healthcare Research and Quality; publication No. 01-E032, contract No. 290-97-0018; Nov 2001.

North American Menopause Society. Menopause: Definitions and Epidemiology. Available at www.menopause.org. Accessed August 2005.

North American Menopause Society. *Menopause Core Curriculum Study Guide,* 2nd ed. Cleveland, OH: The North American Menopause Society; 2002.

North American Menopause Society. Treatment of menopause-associated vasomotor symptoms: position statement of the North American Menopause Society. *Menopause* 2004;11:11–33.

Obermayer-Pietsch BM, Bonelli CM, Walter DE, et al. Genetic predisposition for adult lactose intolerance and relation to diet, bone density, and bone fractures. *J Bone Miner Res* 2004;19:42–47.

Orr-Walker BJ, Evans MC, Ames RW, et al. The effect of past use of the injectable contraceptive depot medroxyprogesterone acetate on bone mineral density in normal post-menopausal women. *Clin Endocrinol (Oxf)* 1998;49:615–618.

Otto F, Thormell AP, Crompton T, et al. CBFA1, a candidate gene for the cleidocranial dysplasia syndrome, is essential for osteoblast formation and bone development. *Cell* 1997;89:765–771.

Phipps KR, Orwoll ES, Mason JD, Cauley JA. Community water fluoridation, bone mineral density, and fractures: prospective study of effects in older women. *BMJ* 2000;321:860–864.

Powels TJ, Hickish T, Kanis JA, Ashley S. Effect of tamoxifen on bone mineral density measured by dual-energy x-ray absorptiometry in healthy premenopausal and postemenopausal women. *J Clin Oncol* 1996;14:78–84.

Prince RL, Devine A, Dhaliwal SS, Dick IM. Effects of calcium supplementation on clinical fracture and bone structure: results of a 5-year, double-blind, placebo-controlled trial in elderly women. *Arch Intern Med* Apr 24 2006;166(8):869–875.

Rauch F, Glorieux FH. Osteogenesis imperfecta. *Lancet* 2004;363:1377–1385.

Ray NF, Chan JK, Thamer M, Melton LJ 3rd. Medical expenditures for the treatment of osteoporotic fractures in the United States in 1995: report from the National Osteoporosis Foundation. *J Bone Miner Res* 1997;12:24–35.

Recker R, Stakkestad JA, Chesnut CH 3rd, et al. Insufficiently dosed intravenous ibandronate injections are associated with suboptimal antifracture efficacy in postmenopausal osteoporosis. *Bone* May 2004;34(5):890–899.

Recommendations for the prevention and treatment of glucocorticoid-induced osteoporosis: 2001 update. American College of Rheumatology Ad Hoc Committee on Glucocorticoid-Induced Osteoporosis. *Arthritis Rheum* Jul 2001;44:1496–1503.

Reid IR, Brown JP, Burckhardt P, et al. Intravenous zoledronic acid in postmenopausal women with low bone mineral density. *N Engl J Med* 2002;346:653–661.

Reginster JY, Seeman E, De Vernejoul MC, et al. Strontium ranelate reduces the risk of nonvertebral fractures in postmenopausal women with osteoporosis: Treatment of Peripheral Osteoporosis (TROPOS) study. *J Clin Endocrinol Metab* 2005;90:2816–2822.

Rejnmark L. et al. Statins decrease bone turnover in postmenopausal women: a cross-sectional study. *Eur J Clin Invest* 2002;32:581–589.

Rittmaster RS, Bolognese M, Ettinger MP, et al. Enhancement of bone mass in osteoporotic women with parathyroid hormone followed by alendronate. *J Clin Endocrinol Metab* 2000; 85(6):2129–2134.

Riggs BL, Melton LJ 3rd. The worldwide problem of osteoporosis: insights afforded by epidemiology. *Bone* 1995;17(Suppl 5):505S–511S.

Rizzoli R, Burlet N, Cahall D, et al. Osteonecrosis of the jaw and bisphosphonate treatment for osteoporosis. *Bone* May 2008; 42(5):841–847.

Robbins J, Hirsch C, Whitmer R, Cauley J, Harris T. The association of bone mineral density and depression in an older population. *J Am Geriatr Soc* 2001;49(6):732–6.

Ronkin S, Northington R, Baracat E, et al. Endometrial effects of bazedoxifene acetate, a novel selective estrogen receptor modulator, in postmenopausal women. *Obstet Gynecol.* Jun 2005;105(6):1397–1404.

Roos EM, Dahlberg L. Positive effects of moderate exercise on glycosaminoglycan content in knee cartilage: a four-month, randomized, controlled trial in patients at risk of osteoarthritis. *Arthritis & Rheumatism* 2005; 52:11:3507–3514.

Rosen CJ, Hochberg MC, Bonnick SL, et al. Treatment with once-weekly alendronate 70 mg compared with once-weekly risedronate 35 mg in women with postmenopausal osteoporosis: a randomized double-blind study. *J Bone Miner Res* 2005;20:141–151.

Ruggiero SL, Mehrotra B, Rosenberg TJ, Engroff SL. Osteonecrosis of the jaw associated with the use of bisphosphonates: a review of 63 cases. *J Oral Maxillofac Surg* May 2004;62(5):527–534.

Saag KG, Emkey R, Schnitzer TJ, et al. Alendronate for the prevention and treatment of glucocorticoid-induced osteoporosis. Glucocorticoid-Induced Osteoporosis Intervention Study Group. *N Engl J Med* 1998;339:292–299.

Salkeld G, Cameron ID, Cumming RG, et al. Quality of life related to fear of falling and hip fracture in older women: a time trade off study. *BMJ* 2000;320:341–346.

Salpeter SR, Walsh JM, Greyber E, et al. Mortality associated with hormone replacement therapy in younger and older women: a meta-analysis. *J Gen Intern Med* 2004;19:791–804.

Sato Y, Honda Y, Iwamoto J, et al. Effect of folate and mecobalamin on hip fractures in patients with stroke: a randomized controlled trial. *JAMA* 2005;293:1082–1088.

Schettler AE, Gustafson EM. Osteoporosis prevention starts in adolescence. *J Am Acad Nurse Pract* Jul 2004;16(7): 274–282.

Schoofs MW, van der Klift M, Hofman A, et al. Thiazide diuretics and the risk for hip fracture. *Ann Intern Med* 2003;139:476–482.

Schull PD. *Nursing Spectrum Drug Handbook.* King of Prussia, PA: Nursing Spectrum; 2005.

Appendix B

Sedlak CA, Doheny MO, Estok PJ, Zeller RA, Winchell J. DXA, health beliefs, and osteoporosis prevention behaviors. *J Aging Health* Oct 2007;19(5):742–756.

Shane E, Goldring S, Christakos S, et al. Osteonecrosis of the jaw: more research needed. *J Bone Miner Res* Oct 2006;21(10):1503–1505.

Shin MH, Holmes MD, Hankinson SE, et al. Intake of dairy products, calcium, and vitamin D and risk of breast cancer. *J Natl Cancer Inst* 2002;94:1301–1311.

Sinaki M, Mikkelsen BA. Postmenopausal spinal osteoporosis: flexion versus extension exercises. *Arch Phys Med Rehabil* 1984;65:593–596.

Siris ES, Miller PD, Barrett-Connor E, et al. Identification and fracture outcomes of undiagnosed low bone mineral density in postmenopausal women: results from the National Osteoporosis Risk Assessment. *JAMA* 2001;286:2815–2822.

Smith MR. Diagnosis and management of treatment-related osteoporosis in men with prostate carcinoma. *Cancer* 2003;97(Suppl 3):789–795.

Stenson WF, Newberry R, Lorenz R, et al R. Increased prevalence of celiac disease and need for routine screening among patients with osteoporosis. *Arch Intern Med* 2005;165: 393–399.

Steptoe A, Wardle J, Marmot M. Positive affect and health-related neuroendocrine, cardiovascular, and inflammatory processes. *Proc Natl Acad Sci USA* 2005;102:6508–6512.

Stuenkel CA. Top ten menopause stories of 2007. *Menopause Management* Jan/Feb 2008;17(1):10–21.

Sunyecz JA, Weisman SM. The role of calcium in osteoporosis drug therapy. *J Womens Health (Larchmt)* 2005;14:180–192.

The American Heritage Stedman's Medical Dictionary. Boston: Houghton Mifflin;1995.

The Merck Manual of Geriatrics, 3rd Edition. 1995–2005. Accessed 2005. Available at: http://www.merck.com/ mrkshared/mmg/home.jsp.

Tosteson AN, Melton LJ 3rd, Dawson-Hughes B, et al. Cost-effective osteoporosis treatment thresholds: the United States perspective. *Osteoporos Int* 2008;19(4):437–447.

Tucker K. Abstract SA330. American Society for Bone and Mineral Research 26th Annual Meeting; Presented October 2, 2004.

U.S. Department of Health and Human Services. *Bone Health and Osteoporosis: A Report of the Surgeon General*. Rockville,

MD: U.S. Department of Health and Human Services, Office of the Surgeon General; 2004.

van Meurs JBJ, Dhonukshe-Rutten RAM, Pluijm SMF, et al. Homocysteine levels and the risk of osteoporotic fracture. *N Engl J Med* 2004;350:2033–2041.

van Schoor NM, Smit JH, Twisk JW, et al. Prevention of hip fractures by external hip protectors: a randomized controlled trial. *JAMA* 2003;289:1957–1962.

Venes D (ed.). *Taber's Cyclopedic Medical Dictionary*, 20th ed. Philadelphia, PA: FA Davis;2005.

Viereck V, Grundker C, Blaschke S, et al. Phytoestrogen genistein stimulates the production of osteoprotegerin by human trabecular osteoblasts. *J Cell Biochem* 2002;84:725–735.

Wardlaw GM. Putting body weight and osteoporosis into perspective. *Am J Clin Nutr* 1996;63(Suppl):433S–436S.

Wasnich RD, Bagger YZ, Hosking DJ, et al. Changes in bone density and turnover after alendronate or estrogen withdrawal. *Menopause* 2004;11(Pt 1):622–630.

Wetli HA, Brenneisen R, Tschudi I, et al. A gamma-glutamyl peptide isolated from onion (*Allium cepa L.*) by bioassay-guided fractionation inhibits resorption activity of osteoclasts. *J Agric Food Chem* 2005;53:3408–3414.

Wolf SL, Barnhart HX, Kutner NG, et al. Reducing frailty and falls in older persons: an investigation of Tai Chi and computerized balance training. Atlanta FICSIT Group. Frailty and Injuries: Cooperative Studies of Intervention Techniques. *J Am Geriatr Soc* 1996;44:489–497.

Woodson GC. Risk factors for osteoporosis in postmenopausal African-American women. *Curr Med Res Opin* 2004;20:1681–1687.

World Health Organization. WHO FRAX technical report. http://www.shef.ac.uk/FRAX/. Accessed May 22, 2009.

World Health Organization. *WHO Scientific Group on the Assessment of Osteoporosis at Primary Health Care Level: Summary Meeting Report.* Brussels, Belgium: WHO Press, Geneva, Switzerland; May 5-7, 2004. 2007.

Wu K, Willett WC, Fuchs CS, et al. Calcium intake and risk of colon cancer in women and men. *J Natl Cancer Inst* 2002;94:437–446.

Yaffe K, Krueger K, Cummings SR, et al. Effect of raloxifene on prevention of dementia and cognitive impairment in older women: the Multiple Outcomes of Raloxifene Evaluation (MORE) randomized trial. *Am J Psychiatry* 2005; 162:683–690.

Glossary

Aerobic exercise: Type of activity intended to strengthen the heart, such as running, cycling, or brisk walking, by increasing your breathing and heart rate; helps the body to burn off fat and control cholesterol.

Alternative therapies: Therapies that are used in place of conventional Western medical therapies; includes massage, visualization, naturopathic medicine, and acupuncture, among others.

Alzheimer's disease: Degenerative brain disorder that gradually causes disorientation, confusion, and memory loss.

Amenorrhea: Absence of menstruation for 3 months or more.

Anabolic agent: Medication, steroid hormone, or substance intended to build bone; examples are Forteo (teriperatide) and testosterone.

Anorexia nervosa: A disorder characterized by fear of becoming obese, thinking the body is larger than it really is, severe weight loss, and an aversion to food. Once thought to only affect teenage girls, it is now recognized in women of all ages and rarely in men.

Antiresorptive agents: Medications and substances that decrease bone resorption (bone breakdown).

Biochemical marker: Substances found in blood and urine that can be tested to determine the rate of bone turnover.

Bioidentical: Refers to hormones manufactured in a laboratory, usually from wild yam or soy, which have the exact same chemical makeup as the hormones made in the body; also termed "natural" hormones.

Bisphosphonates: A group of antiresorptive agents, such as Fosamax,

Boniva, and Actonel, which slow the rate at which bone is broken down.

Body mass index (BMI): A measurement of body size that includes both height and weight. It is calculated by dividing your weight (in pounds) by your squared height (in inches), multiplied by 704.5.

Bone mass: The volume, density, or quantity of bone.

Bone mineral density (BMD) tests: Safe, painless, and noninvasive tests to evaluate bone mineral density.

Bone modeling: A process that takes place in childhood and adolescence in which new bone is developed at one site and old bone is destroyed at another site. For healthy bones during bone growth, the amount of new bone being formed should exceed the amount of old bone being broken down.

Bone remodeling: A process that occurs after peak bone mass is reached in early adulthood. Bone forming cells respond to the activity of the bone breakdown cells. When bone formation does not keep pace with bone breakdown, osteoporosis occurs.

Bone turnover: The process of breaking down bone and forming new bone in its place, a process that occurs throughout life. When bone is growing (during childhood through early adulthood) new formation exceeds breakdown; later in life breakdown exceeds formation.

Bulimia: An eating disorder that usually includes episodes of binge eating (eating very large amounts of food) and purging (forcing vomiting or diarrhea to get food out of the system).

Calcitonin: A hormone naturally secreted by the thyroid gland that makes the osteoclasts less active, allowing for more bone formation to take place.

Calcitriol: A hormone resulting from the conversion of vitamin D by liver and kidney enzymes to aid in balancing the activity of the osteoclasts and osteoblasts.

Calcium: A mineral necessary for the production and function of bone. It is removed from bone when blood levels of calcium become low; also vital for functioning of nerves and muscles. Calcium must be consumed daily and is found in many dairy products, certain vegetables, fortified products, and supplements.

Cartilage: Rubbery connective tissue that is found in joints and the outer ear.

Central bones: Bones that are found in the main or central areas of the body, such as the hips, vertebrae, and spine. These bones provide the best measures for determining bone mineral density.

Central testing: Usually DXA or QCT bone density tests of the hip, upper thigh, or spine.

Collagen: A protein substance used by osteoblasts to make new bone and keep teeth strong. Also found in connective tissue such as skin, tendons, and ligaments throughout the body.

Complementary therapies: Therapies that are used in addition to conventional, Western medical treatments or interventions.

Conjugated equine estrogen: The most common form of estrogen used in hormone therapy (HT), extracted from the urine of pregnant mares.

Contrast dye: A dye that is given orally or intravenously for the purposes of focusing certain types of imaging tests; should not be taken within 2 weeks before having a bone mineral density test.

Cortical bone: Hard outer shell of bone responsible for bone strength.

Cortisol: A steroid hormone secreted by the adrenal glands necessary for bone growth. Too much cortisol can cause bone loss.

Dementia: Condition marked by memory loss, lack of ability to attend to personal care, personality changes, impaired reasoning, and bouts of disorientation.

DHEA (dehydroepiandrosterone): A precursor to testosterone secreted by the adrenal glands and ovaries; in supplement form, made from steroid molecules extracted from wild yam, an herb.

Dialysis: Process by which impurities and toxic substances are removed from the body either by filtering blood through a machine or infusing fluids into the abdominal cavity that remove wastes; required for those who do not have adequately functioning kidneys.

Disability: A physical or mental impairment that causes inability to perform normal or routine activities.

Dowager's hump: see Kyphosis.

DXA (dual-energy x-ray absorptiometry): A test that measures bone mineral density in the hip, upper thigh, and spine. DXA tests use a particular form of x-ray imaging that is analyzed through a computer to give results in the terms of T-scores and Z-scores; gold standard for measuring bone loss and diagnosing osteoporosis.

Elemental calcium: The calcium that your body absorbs and uses.

Endocrinologist: Physician who specializes in the care of people with hormone disorders such as diabetes, thyroid problems, and osteoporosis.

Endometriosis: A painful condition characterized by the abnormal presence of endometrial (uterine lining) tissue outside the uterus, such as on the ovary, colon, or bladder.

Estrogen: Known as a female sex hormone although it is also found in men in small amounts; primarily secreted by the ovary in response to follicle stimulating hormone (FSH) and is also made in body tissues in both men and women. Estrogens used in hormone therapy (HT) can be manufactured using certain plants or from pregnant mare's urine.

Estrogen agonist/antagonist: Antiresorptive medications such as Evista that help to reduce bone loss by their positive estrogenic effects; formerly known as selective estrogen receptor modulators or SERMs.

Glossary

Estrogen receptor positive cancer: Type of cancer that is estrogen dependent or has receptors for estrogen.

Estrogen therapy (ET): Estrogen-containing products that are used in the treatment of perimenopausal and menopausal symptoms. Estrogen taken by itself for the treatment of menopausal symptoms is also called MHT (menopause hormone therapy).

Extension: Straightening a flexed limb.

Flexion: A bending motion of any joint.

Folate: A vitamin needed for new cell development; helps reduce levels of homocysteine, a substance associated with osteoporotic fractures, heart disease, and stroke; also reduces risks for breast and colon cancer; also called folic acid. A vitamin found in fruits, vegetables, and low-fat dairy products and lowers homocysteine levels; a substance associated with osteoporotic fractures.

Fracture: To break, splinter, or crack a bone.

Fragility fracture: Term used to describe a fracture that occurs with very little trauma or force and from a height that is usually not great enough to cause broken bones, usually indicating that the bone is weak. Also called an osteoporotic fracture.

Frozen bone: Speculated to be a potential concern in individuals taking combinations of osteoporosis medications. While the medications increase bone mass, the bone quality may not be as good, resulting in bone that is more brittle rather than stronger.

Glucocorticoid-induced osteoporosis: Osteoporosis caused by taking glucocorticoids (commonly called steroids), a class of medications taken for their anti-inflammatory effects on illnesses such as rheumatoid arthritis, asthma, lupus, and Crohn's disease.

Gluten intolerance: Allergy to wheat, which occurs in celiac disease. Can cause intestinal absorption problems.

Growth hormone: Hormone secreted by the pituitary gland and especially important for bone growth during puberty.

Gynecology clinician (GYN): A nurse practitioner, midwife, physician assistant, or physician who specializes in the practice of gynecology, the health care of women; often focused primarily on their reproductive organs.

Half-life: Time it takes the body to metabolize or inactivate half of the amount of a medication that was taken.

Hip protector: A protective pad worn over the hip.

Homocysteine: A substance associated with fractures due to osteoporosis as well as heart disease; can be reduced by eating a diet high in folic acid (e.g., green leafy vegetables and fruits) or by taking vitamins B_6 and B_{12}.

Hot flashes: Sensations of heat, occurring during perimenopause and often well into postmenopause, that begin at the head and spread over the entire body; occurs with an increase in lutenizing hormone. Is not a health hazard, may be accompanied by sweating, and can cause significant discomfort or interfere with sleep.

Hypogonadism: Inadequate testicular or ovarian function most commonly causing low levels of testosterone.

Hysterectomy: Removal of the uterus.

Idiopathic ovarian insufficiency: The loss of ovarian function (and therefore fertility) in a woman under the age of 40, resulting in menopause. It is usually associated with other health conditions and can sometimes be temporary. Also called premature ovarian failure.

Induced menopause: Permanent menopause that is not natural; can be caused as a result of removal of the ovaries (surgical), chemotherapy, or radiation to the pelvis.

Injection: Given into the muscle, fat tissue, or vein using a needle with a syringe attached.

Insulin: A hormone secreted by the pancreas and important for the body's ability to use carbohydrates and sugar.

Isoflavone: A type of phytoestrogen found most notably in soy and red clover.

Kyphoplasty: A surgical procedure used to relieve pain of VCFs, which combines vertebroplasty and angioplasty by placing a balloon in the fractured vertebra and filling it with a cement-like substance.

Kyphosis: A deformity of the spine that develops when the front edges of the bones of the spine collapse due to osteoporosis and fractures; also called "dowager's hump."

Lactose intolerance: Occurs when the small intestine does not make enough lactase, the enzyme required to break down the lactose (milk sugar) in milk products before they enter the large intestine; can cause bloating, pain, gas, and diarrhea.

Leptin: A hormone found in fat cells that affects bone growth.

Ligaments: Tough bands that connect bones to each other.

Long bones: The larger bones of the legs (femur, tibia, fibula) and arms (humerus, ulna, radius).

Lysine: An amino acid that strengthens collagen in bone formation.

Magnesium: A mineral important for hardening of bone.

Menopause: The specific point in time occurring after 12 consecutive months without a menstrual period that does not have another identifiable cause such as illness or medications.

MHT (menopause hormone therapy): Hormone therapy (HT) was changed to MHT to distinguish it from other types of hormone therapy that are not given to alleviate the symptoms of menopause. See estrogen therapy.

Night sweats: Sweating that occurs at night resulting from hot flashes during perimenopause and postmenopause.

Obesity: Condition of being severely overweight based on body mass index greater than 30 and associated with many health problems; a leading cause of death in the United States.

Orthopedist: A physician who specializes in the treatment and surgery of bone and joint disorders.

Osteoarthritis: Inflammation and stiffness of the joints that usually occurs in older persons as a result of deterioration of the cartilage around the joints.

Osteoblasts: Cells that cause bone formation.

Osteocalcin: A protein that is part of the bone remodeling cycle.

Osteoclasts: Cells that cause bone breakdown.

Osteomalacia: A softening of bones caused by vitamin D deficiency because of diet or ailments that impair normal vitamin D absorption or use; causes bone pain, leg deformities, and fractures; sometimes called adult rickets.

Osteonecrosis of the jaw: Deterioration of jaw bone associated with tooth loss, local infection, and delayed healing; leads to death of local jaw bone tissue.

Osteopenia: A condition in which there is low bone mass or low bone density, but not to the same degree as osteoporosis. Osteopenia means bones (osteo) are lacking (penia). T-score is between –1.0 and –2.5.

Osteoporosis: The most common bone disease, in which bones become less dense, lose strength, and are more likely to break (fracture). Osteoporosis means bones (osteo) with holes (porosis). T-score is lower than –2.5.

Oversuppression: Occurs when bone turnover is suppressed to such a high extent that bone quality may be compromised; associated with "frozen bone."

Paget's disease: Causes large, deformed bones due to the excessive breakdown and formation of bone. Although totally unrelated to osteoporosis, it can occur with osteoporosis in the same bones.

Panoramic x-ray: A type of radiography, usually of teeth and surrounding bones such as the jawbone.

Parathyroid hormone (PTH): A hormone secreted by the parathyroid glands that assists in the regulation of calcium by promoting the absorption of calcium from the intestine and reducing the loss of calcium through urine excretion. Also the active ingredient in Forteo, a medication and anabolic agent used to treat osteoporosis.

pDXA (peripheral dual-energy x-ray absorptiometry): Uses the same technology as the DXA but measures bone density in the wrist, forearm, finger, or heel.

Peak bone mass: The highest amount of bone present in the human body, usually obtained by early adulthood.

Pedometer: A small gadget that measures the number of footsteps taken.

Periodontal disease: Disease of the gums, tissues, and bone supporting teeth.

Peripheral bone mineral density testing: Bone mineral density tests of the non-central bones, usually heel, wrist, forearm, or fingers.

Peripheral limbs: The outer areas of the body, including hands, forearms, wrists, lower leg, and feet.

Phosphorus: A mineral important for the formation of bone and teeth.

Phytoestrogens: Weak, estrogen-like substances that are in plants. Can be eaten in whole foods, such as soy, or extracted from red clover in the form of isoflavones and made into supplements.

Pilates: A type of activity for muscles that promotes strength and flexibility; developed by Joseph Pilates, this group of exercises can be done by yourself or in a class.

Placebo: An inactive substance that contains no medication or active ingredient; to be given to participants in a clinical trial to determine the effectiveness of a specific treatment or medication.

Plantar fasciitis: An inflammation of the connective tissue of the bottom of the foot, which can cause severe pain.

Postmenopause: The time following menopause during which estrogen loss is the major cause of osteoporosis in women past midlife.

pQCT (peripheral quantitative computed tomography): Type of radiography that uses the same technology as the QCT but measures bone density in the forearm or wrist; primarily used in research.

Premature menopause: Permanent (usually natural) menopause occurring in women younger than 40 years of age; also refers to women who have induced or surgical menopause.

Premature ovarian failure: The loss of ovarian function (and therefore fertility) in a woman under the age of 40, resulting in menopause. It is usually associated with other health conditions and can sometimes be temporary. Also called idiopathic ovarian insufficiency.

Prescription medication: An instruction from a health care professional who is licensed to provide written authorization of medications or devices to be issued by a pharmacy.

Primary osteoporosis: Type of osteoporosis related to age that affects women more severely and earlier than men.

QCT (quantitative computed tomography): Type of radiography that uses CT scan technology to measure the bone density in the spine.

QUS (quantitative ultrasound): Type of radiography that uses sound wave technology to test the bone density of the heel, wrist, tibia bone in the leg, and fingers.

RA (radiographic absorptiometry): Conventional x-ray with software and scanning equipment used to measure bone density of the middle bones of the hand.

Radiogrammetry: Like radiographic absorptiometry, an imaging technique that uses conventional x-rays by comparing the bone density of the two bones in the hand.

Resistive exercise: Type of activity that pushes and pulls muscles to strengthen them; examples are swimming, biking, and weight-lifting.

Resorption: Process by the osteoclasts of breaking down bone.

Rheumatologist: Physician who specializes in the care of people with disorders related to joints, bones, tendons, and muscles. Unlike a surgeon, does not perform surgery on joints and bones.

Salpingo-oophorectomy: Removal of fallopian tube and ovary; *bilateral* means both fallopian tubes and both ovaries are removed.

Secondary osteoporosis: Osteoporosis at any age resulting from illnesses, conditions, or medications that cause bone loss.

Sedentary lifestyle: A way of living that involves little or no exercise.

Severe osteoporosis: A T-score lower than −2.5 plus the presence of one or more fragility fractures.

Sex hormones: A chemical substance formed in one organ or part of the body that can alter the function or structure of another organ, tissue, or various numbers of them; examples are estrogen, testosterone, and progesterone, which stimulate bone growth.

Standard deviation: A mathematical measure that indicates how far or how near something is to the mean (average).

Supplements: Additional doses of vitamins, minerals, or other dietary substances; usually taken to enhance diet to get the recommended amount for your age, gender, and medical conditions.

SXA (single energy x-ray absorptiometry): Type of radiograph where the bone mineral density test is done on the wrist or heel while the body part is submerged in water.

Tai chi: A form of exercise that combines meditation and flexibility training.

Testosterones: A steroid hormone formed by the testes in males and, to a far lesser degree, by the ovary and adrenal glands in women; responsible for male characteristics such as a deep voice and facial hair; is important for normal sexual development and function as well as normal bone development in both men and women.

Thyroid hormones: Secreted by the thyroid gland, these natural chemicals regulate the body's metabolism and help to control the rate of bone remodeling; too much can cause bone destruction.

Total hysterectomy: Although technically only refers to removal of the uterus, "total" is sometimes used to refer to removal of the uterus, ovaries, and fallopian tubes.

Trabecular bone: Connective spongy tissue of bone, particularly of the central and long bones. Provides strength and integrity, houses bone marrow, produces blood products, and provides the surface used for the exchange of calcium and phosphorus.

T-score: A positive or negative number representing the number of standard deviations that is calculated based on a comparison between your bone mineral density with that of healthy young adults. T-scores between −1.0 and −2.5 indicate osteopenia; T-scores lower than −2.5 indicate osteoporosis.

Vasomotor symptoms: Symptoms resulting from irregular functioning of the part of the brain that controls body heat, usually experienced as hot flashes and sweats that may or may not be followed by feeling cold or chilled.

Vertebrae: Individual bones of the spine. Fractures of these bones are the most common fractures in people with osteoporosis.

Vertebral compression fracture (VCF): A fracture of the body of a vertebra (spine bone) that collapses it and makes it thinner and weaker. Usually results from osteoporosis but can also result from complications of cancer or some injuries.

Vertebral fracture: See vertebral compression fracture.

Vertebroplasty: A nonsurgical procedure that involves injecting a cement-like substance into the fractured vertebra to stabilize it and relieve pain.

Vitamin: One of a group of organic substances, present in minute amounts in natural foodstuffs, that are essential to normal metabolism; insufficient amounts in the diet may cause deficiency diseases.

Vitamin A: Plays an essential role in growing healthy bones by helping to regulate osteoclast and osteoblast activities in bone modeling and remodeling; too much of it can actually damage your bones.

Vitamin B$_6$: Indirectly helps with bone development by lowering levels of homocysteine.

Vitamin C: Important for bone development because of its role in making collagen.

Vitamin D: Also known as calciferol, which is actually a hormone; a nutrient important for absorbing and regulating calcium and phosphorus levels. Sunlight, fortified products, or supplements are necessary in order to get the required amount of daily vitamin D.

Vitamin K: Aids in the production of osteocalcin; also important for the blood's ability to clot; helps to prevent calcium from being removed from bone. Insufficient vitamin K can lead to hip fractures.

Weight-bearing exercise: Type of activity that places weight on certain bones; necessary for bone growth; examples are walking, dancing, and stair-climbing.

Yoga: A group of breathing exercises and movements intended to improve flexibility and strength, and bring about tranquility.

Z-score: Matches your bone mineral density with individuals of the same age, gender, and ethnicity, but is more helpful in evaluating children and premenopausal women. Very low Z-scores may mean that you have secondary osteoporosis.

Index

Index

Index

Index

Index